KEITH'S INSPIRATIONAL STORY
NEGOTIATING WITH CANCER

SURVIVE

REVIVE

THRIVE

Maryla Mary Storm

Keith's Inspirational Story Negotiating With Cancer

Survive, Revive, Thrive

First Edition

Edited by: Elizabeth Ridley, Martha Lang, and Kiersten Vannest.

Cover art by: www.fiverr.com/art_infinity

Formatting by: www.fiverr.com/cmgraphicshub

DEDICATION

To my loving, dancing husband, Keith, whose inspiration lives on,
NOW and FOREVER!

CONTENTS

ACKNOWLEDGMENTS

Writing this book has been one of the most challenging jobs in my life. But at the same time, it has been most satisfying and cathartic. Of course, without further ADIEU (I say this because of my husband's mother's French sayings), I must thank my ever-faithful Superman of my entire life, Keith. For without Keith's long cancer journey and his trials and triumphs, miracles of miracles, and his own penning part of this book, there would not be a book

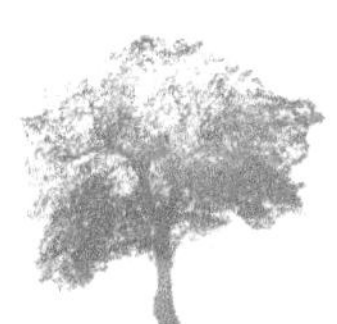

INTRODUCTION

"You never know how strong you are until being strong is the only choice you have." *(Bob Marley)*

My dearest husband, Keith, was definitely the strongest man I ever knew. Maybe not strong in the sense of his ability to lift a house with his right arm—but producing in the way of a formidable Superman-type nevertheless.

"Whatever doesn't kill you, makes you stronger." Paraphrased quote by Friedrich Nietzsche (1888). This statement was, without a doubt, true in Keith's case. After all, Keith had survived more than eleven years. For eleven years, he lived while thriving with stage 4 colon cancer. Even though the doctors only gave Keith a few months at most to live his last days here on earth. All that after already enduring a tough family life. I figured that Keith had learned and earned to be a strong survivor.

Keith wanted to be like his idol, John Wayne—invincible, strong, able to fight the fight, and a "True Grit" type of person. So, he strapped on his imaginary cancer-fighting guns and went to work. Time after time, Keith continued to fight the fight, year after year. He fought with grit and courageous determination. Why? Because he wanted to continue living no matter what.

About a year into Keith's cancer journey, we began referring to Keith as Superman, after the DC comic legend. Because at every turn of his cancer journey, Keith's tenaciousness and strength showed the way to handle living with cancer. You ought to read about the times we thought Keith even glowed in the dark! (read more in the Y90 sections).

Keith had the fiercest instinct to persevere and survive! He certainly squeezed every bit of dynamism out of life. Never in my life had I known anyone going through so much for so long while fighting cancer—wanting to live the fullest life at the same time.

Keith had endured so many surgeries, procedures, ordeals, never-ending chemotherapy, and other infusions. Yet, during all those years, he continued to stay optimistic about continuing with living to the max. It was Keith's ever-flowing positive, optimistic attitude that aided him to take a two-month sentence and stretch that for more than eleven years. He could have wallowed in self-pity and lain in bed, and given up. No doubt he would've been gone quickly. But he wanted more. He wanted more days, and he wanted more nights here as a human being living in the here and now.

So, with determination, what I witnessed during Keith's cancer journey was a fighter with great courage using power through positive thinking plus a loving, giving gratitude attitude. Keith was all that plus more.

Along with positive thoughts, Keith's sustaining life, without a doubt, happened because of all of the great doctors and their skills. Keith also engaged in many complementary modalities of healing.

Keith garnered inspiring resilience. Somehow, he was often able to recuperate quickly after most of the difficulties of his cancer journey. Keith constantly amazed me (and others) through the years by getting out on the dance floor days after receiving chemotherapy infusions. When the doctors told Keith that he would be out of commission after surgery for six weeks, he would usually be back at activities within three weeks. Keith did not want to miss out on a moment he could capture. He had a purpose of living and finding happiness where he could and when he was able.

Someone pointed out to me that part of Keith's inspirational will to continue thriving while fighting cancer was because of me. I had not thought of that before. After all, I was doing my duty of attending my husband. Another person told me straight out that Keith did not want to leave me at all! I didn't want him to go, either. I know I helped Keith every day to support him in ridding his body of cancer. The devotion between Keith and me was undeniable.

I had often overheard people query Keith about how he kept surviving for so many years. Keith's varied responses were always with a positive attitude. He would talk about how God's assistance, the doctors' support, and my help would get him through one step at a time.

I figured that because Keith and I had already made our way through callous times so far in life, we were combat-ready for Keith's cancer. No question about it, our life experiences helped us develop into stronger individuals. We progressed forward once the cancer was in our crosshairs. The two of us discovered that we were Stronger Together! And staying Strong Together would be needed for the journey ahead—taking out the cancer!

We always put God first and foremost. It was the glue that held our marriage in concert. We were proud of our marriage, our union, our partnership. We worked hard at our meaningful collaboration. We lived by this quote: "LOVE NEVER GIVES UP." (1 Corinthians 13:7)

Knowing full well that Keith needed our durable union in the fight of his life, staying together was imperative. I never once wanted to give up and leave Keith to fight alone. We had heard of couples splitting when faced with massive trials such as cancer. But I sure could not even imagine how anyone could just walk away from a person they are supposed to love (until death do us part).

Keith relied upon and had a big belief in his faith, along with his deep connection to HOPE. He never gave up the Hope that he would live long enough that a new cancer treatment would evolve and eradicate his cancer once and for all. His life was all about living his faith and knowing there was always HOPE. Because HOPE NEVER DIES!

Keith was courageously inspirational because he wanted to live and thrive instead of simply surviving the cancer ordeal. We called that Carpe Diem. Keith and I seized every opportunity, every potential day we could, so that Keith would be able to live the fullest possible life for whatever time he had to come. Each day we woke, Keith would proclaim it a Carpe Diem Day if he didn't have a procedure, test, surgery, or a therapy on the agenda. Even if he did not feel up to par, he would still pull himself up and out because he knew he would feel better and better once he got out there and did something. The simple act of taking a walk at the beach breathed new life into both of us. Getting out into nature, hearing the water and the waves hitting the sand, and just simply being in the sun regenerated Keith (and me).

Of course, part of our Carpe Diem days worked into weekends and even weeks. Keith was the one who talked about and pre-planned most trips. A lot of our trips were for dancing. Dancing trips and getaways, short or long, all filled Keith (and me) with an abundance of JOY! We were constantly revving up the JOY!

Such a motivating person to everyone was my Keith. It was because of his inspiration that I wrote this book. Long ago, during his early cancer time, Keith began writing about his cancer journey. Of course, he would share some of his experiences with others, and his amazed friends kept telling him, "You gotta write a book!" With that,

Keith would always turn to me and smile. He knew it was on my to-do list. For years, after saying prayers for Keith at the end of a busy day, as I lay there waiting for sleep, I would often plan Keith's book in my mind.

Keith always wanted his writings, his journal, to be published to help others. He also wanted me to share with everyone all of the methods he used that assisted him through every inch of every day to live another day to its fullest.

Whether it be for a newbie just notified about their own cancer and wanting to improve their odds, or perhaps a loved one of a cancer patient in search of the light at the end of the tunnel, Keith always hoped to show the positive way to live the NEW normal as a cancer-fighting person.

Now you know a bit about Keith, and I have touched upon some of the ameliorating factors that kept Keith alive for so long. It is my belief that God's (and the) Universe's plan all along was to keep Keith here on earth long enough to be an inspiration to people everywhere. Keith was here to teach us all lessons. Lessons about attitude, positive thinking, having faith and hope and never giving up, staying strong with true grit, using research and advocacy, and complementary modes of healing for the fight for his life. Plus, lessons of living the fullest life each and every day no matter what.

Going forth, you will find more in-depth information that can be helpful for:

- Spouses with cancer

- Family members with cancer who need guidance and inspiration on how to live with cancer

- People who have a significant other fighting cancer and who they want to help

- Persons with cancer feeling lost

- Someone who has lost a loved one to cancer and need

inspiration for transcending their grief

Along with getting to know Keith and me more, you will learn more about our marriage and how we managed to stay effective together and keep the happiness factor going. You will also be able to read about Keith's cancer treatments, procedures, surgeries, and how Keith used many techniques that helped him get through it all. For those looking for help, Keith has a lot of tips for how he handled nausea and so many other problems, such as what he did about his PICC line and port-a-cath issues and a bit about his nasty ostomy and liver bile bags.

I have included all of what Keith wrote in his chronologically dated journal in this book. Furthermore, I have given great detail to the near-death stroke Keith suffered and the miracle that brought him back to reality and good health. I included this critical passage in Keith's cancer saga so that people can see that sometimes when medical authorities say that "that is all there is," it may not be accurate. Remember this—NEVER GIVE UP!

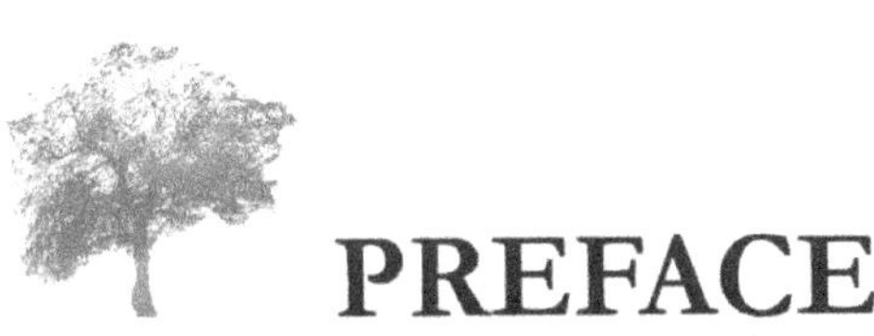

PREFACE

How did Keith last so long living with cancer? I think that was the most-often-asked question about my precious husband. Therein lies the whole truth of why I wrote this teaching memoir story—because people wanted to know. Of course, the rest of the story is that Keith all along thought about helping others. From the start of his journey, he/we often said, "Wow, wish we had help with this," "Wish we knew this before it happened," "Wish we had a warning about that." Keith wished that others would learn from what we learned—How to thrive and not just survive while fighting cancer.

I had been involved with book-writing with others, and when I was young, I loved to read and write stories. So, it was all too natural to fall into helping Keith spread the knowledge that we gained from Keith's experience through his cancer expedition.

For your information, I did not do a lot of research primarily to write this book. You see, from the start I was researching to help save Keith from cancer. I researched everything so that we would have a full understanding every step of the way. After meetings with doctors (and sometimes during a meeting) research would be done and articles and books read, as soon as we returned home. What did the doctor call that word? Yes, and what was the process he talked about? What were the side effects of that chemotherapy or drug? I would jump on the interwebs and learn everything I could. Each report was dissected word by word until we had knowledge that we understood or that we could take to another source to get more definitions. I saved everything along the way. I collected everything in my research folder. Just in case we needed to look at it later, it would easily be at the tip of our fingers.

My research wasn't just for medical terms. I also did research when Dean-O and Pat began their treatments on Keith. Neither of us knew much about the subject of Qigong and Tama-do; therefore, much research was warranted. Tama-do involves sound and color healing and Qigong is effective in improving health and preventing sickness.

Keith also was helped with research when it came to Tai Chi and the other methods he used to help him thrive the long eleven years. Tai-chi is also effective to improve one's health and well-being. We both sincerely believed that because of research and the many systems Keith used, he was able to fully thrive while fighting the evil cancer.

The process of writing this book took a few years after Keith's demise. I had some things underway in my mind that started forming during Keith's last year. But getting them put to paper (not really— typed into the computer) was difficult to accomplish right after Keith's passing. But writing was a healing, powerful way to help process what was happening to me as I figured out my new life without my husband.

I wrote no matter what almost every day. I think it helped me work through the coping process of realizing that he did die. Even when I wrote this preface, I was again astonished that he was gone. By now, in 2022, he has been gone two years. My mind has been clearer than two years ago as the brain fog has melted away. Thankfully.

Going through so much after someone passes and trying to accomplish writing a book was sometimes very daunting. But I never met a challenge I walked away from.

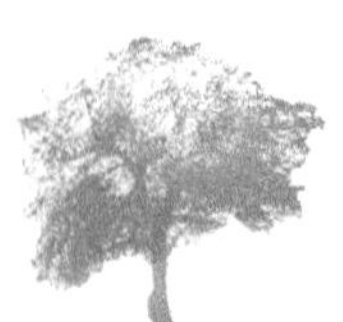

ABOUT KEITH

Lorraine and David Storm's only child, Keith, was born in 1949 in Inglewood, California. Then the family moved back East and around various states following David's jobs.

Keith's childhood growing up was not without problems. Since the family often moved due to his father's work, constant disruption transpired for this youngster. Each time he moved to a new city, Keith met new people, attended a new school, and met new fellow students. Moving around so much and being an only child left Keith incredibly lonely. Oftentimes he played with imaginary friends to keep him company as he drove his toy cars.

The home life problems were all about Keith's mother, Lorraine. She suffered an imbalance (this is what Keith learned), and Lorraine tried her best to take care of Keith. Keith found it safest for him to learn early on to be self-sufficient to be less a problem for his mother. He talked of spending many nights alone in his room playing or reading. So that Keith would be out of the way and not cause problems, he played alone in his room much of the time, making little noise, and did not ask friends to come over. Once he was old enough, he spent much of his time outside or at his friends' homes.

Keith told me stories about one particular happy period in his preteens when he and his family lived just blocks away from Disneyland in Anaheim, California. He befriended someone from school, and because the climate was almost always warm to hot, they spent a lot of time outdoors on their bikes. If anyone knew about Disneyland when they started out, they issued tickets for each ride, and a family would buy a whole booklet of tickets for each person upon entering Disneyland for the day. Each booklet would have so many A-tickets, B-tickets, C-tickets, D-tickets, and the coveted E-tickets for the Matterhorn Bobsleds. Years later, people still use the coveted ticket in describing rides everywhere; "Wow, that was an E-TICKET RIDE!" There would be more A tickets and fewer E-tickets in each pack purchased.

Keith said he and his friend were primarily gifted A and B-tickets. But once in a while, they would get lucky and receive C and D-tickets. Never the winner E-ticket. That's because they were the most popular and always used right away by the ticket purchasers.

It was guaranteed that there would be spare ride tickets at the end of the day for most people. That's because people spent much time standing in line and going on the very fastest and most finest rides. Time ran out for everyone, and there was never time to use those last tickets.

Keith didn't tell me much about how he would end up with the left-over tickets. But I could imagine that family and friends would come to town to visit them and would leave and hand Keith the left-over tickets.

But another part of me thought that he and his friends might have stood at the exit to Disneyland and asked for any left-over tickets as people left.

Keith told me that once they had a bunch of tickets, they rode their bikes to Disneyland, locked them up at the bike racks, and spent the day cashing in on all the left-over tickets. Although they had to go on very little kid rides like the Sleeping Beauty Castle or Alice in Wonderland.

Growing up, Keith went to work as soon as he could at the local gas stations. Since he was a "car" guy, he loved being around cars, pumping gas, checking oil, and wiping windows. He also loved to watch and help the greasers (mechanics) in the garage at the gas station.

At home or with his friends, Keith focused on cars. Tinkering, adjusting this or that, making the hot rods loud with rumbling sounds, then off he and his friends would go on any given night—cruising the beaches, Sunset Strip, Hollywood. Every guy in those days loved to show off their rides and pick up girls for a cruising time.

After following Keith's father's jobs around the country, the family returned to Inglewood in later years, where Keith lettered in varsity track and graduated from Inglewood High School.

Not long after Inglewood High, the Vietnam War ushered Keith quickly to the jungles of Vietnam, the island of Guam, and later Vandenberg Air Force Base, where he worked with bomb munitions (conventional and nuclear).

He was proud to serve in the Air Force. But once he returned home from Vietnam, he was greatly disheartened when people yelled at him and threw eggs at him and the other service members as they arrived at the airport.

After his Air Force tour, Keith followed his father in the high-rise engineering field. After a stretch working with the U.S. Postal Service while obtaining schooling and training, Keith joined the IUOE Local 501 as an Operating Engineer, maintaining high-rise buildings in downtown Los Angeles as well as other southland areas.

It did not take long before Keith achieved Chief Operating Engineer status, working over thirty-six tireless years with his team, winning building of the year awards (BOMA–Building Owners and

Managers Association International).

It is important to report about Keith's father's cancer. David was diagnosed with bone cancer not long before his sixtieth birthday. Keith was close to forty years old at the time. Keith had to watch as his dad's pain became extreme and brutal to handle. Keith told stories of hearing his father's loud, anguished calls for help, and he knew he was in a great deal of horrible pain. After all, men in the family did not reveal many emotions. Keith had his own life, but he was often called to fetch the special pain-relieving ingredients to ease his father's pain. Keith said he would give his dad the unique formula (in liquid form), and the drugs would quickly knock out David's pain and put him to sleep. After a time with the excruciating pain, David passed away just days before his sixtieth birthday. No more pain for Keith's father.

Twenty-five years later, Keith was diagnosed with stage 4 (metastasized to liver and lymph nodes) colon cancer just months before his sixtieth birthday. Of course, it was a déjà vu experience for him, along with visions of his father's cancer and pain coming to the forefront of Keith's mind. He often wondered, out loud to himself and me, "Would I also be in that awful pain my father had to endure? Would I die by my sixtieth birthdate? Would I follow in my father's cancer steps?" Keith was petrified with fright about all of this early on.

However, as I did all along, I gave Keith much love and support to allow him to make the required effort to live another day, another month, another year, year after year.

Now, you must have heard of and seen the famous movie Erin Brockovich? If not, read about it here on her website, https://www.brockovich.com/the-movie/. All about PG & E covering up chromium poisoning the local water supply of a rural city in California and people in the town dying of cancer.

Well, we believe that both Keith and his father suffered this same fate for the same reason: chromium poisoning. Not because they lived in that town. But they unknowingly worked with the cleaning products containing chromium in their jobs.

Why? Because, during their lives, both Keith and his father worked with processing the same job: Both were engineers and cleaned the cooling towers with chromium—no gloves or masks were ever encouraged or used. Of course, we do not have absolute proof and never sought legal advice on the matter. But we couldn't help but wonder after watching the *Brockovich* movie multiple times whether this was the main factor for their cancers.

We also believed that Keith's involvement with munitions bomb material, including nuclear, contributed to the cancer equation. Keith did not inherit the cancer—this we knew for sure. Tests would later reveal this to be true.

It is important to note that Keith not only had his dad's death cross to bear, but he also had to deal with his mother's situation constantly. You see, David placed Keith's mother, Lorraine, in a care center before he passed away. Lorraine had suffered a stroke years earlier and needed constant care. After David's death, Keith saw his mother in person five days a week for most of the rest of her life.

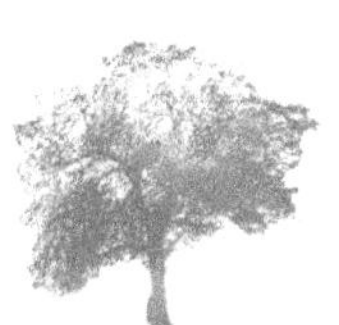

ABOUT MARY

I was born in the 1950s in a dinky old fashion town not too far from my grandparent's farm home in Northern Texas, where tenant farming was the norm. My assiduous grandparents and uncles farmed for the property owners in exchange for rent, food, and a bit of stipend. I have old photos depicting the extreme, harsh conditions they endured farming the food and cotton.

I was born in Texas because my mom had come to her parent's home since there was a hospital nearby. There was not a town or hospital within fifty miles of where my mother and father lived in Wyoming. After I was born, my mom and I stayed at my grandparent's home until my father finished his railroad job in Wyoming. Then, once he arrived, I was old enough to travel to visit relatives. After that, we settled in Bishop, California for my first seven years.

I giggled to myself as I remembered the fun we experienced in Bishop. I was the oldest of the five siblings (three brothers and one sister), with most of us being very close in age (from one to five years) with the exception of the baby who was born when I was fourteen.

Being the most senior of a group of siblings was sometimes fun and other times hard work. The fun would often entail leading my brothers and sisters on a trek down the lane, next to the watering crick, to the blackberry bushes. Mom gave us the job of picking enough berries for a pie. I handed out the containers to collect the berries, and I handed out the instructions. Mother would always run for the camera upon our return. That's because our faces and hands showed a lot of evidence that perhaps we ate more than we placed in the containers. That was the fun that I recollected.

Once we moved to Southern California, what I loved most, as a youngster, was organizing our neighborhood friends and producing small plays, musicals, and puppet shows in our backyard. We used the clothesline for draping sheets for show curtains. We even sold tickets I made with my small rubber printing cubes. Those were fun times and the way children of yesterday learned to work together. By the way, the proceeds for these events (we invited the parents and other friends for a price) went toward a walk to the neighborhood malt shop for all the participants. No one ever fought over what was purchased. Everyone shared. Good ole days!

The hard work of being top of the line, leader of the pack, and mother's helper would stay with me for the rest of my life. It seemed that anywhere and everywhere I was, I would end up leading, handling, overseeing, and taking care of projects and people in my life. Such was the case with my parents and siblings since they always looked to me for guidance. My siblings still do.

Then there were the callous times. While growing up, perhaps at age nine and after, life became complicated when Dad took to alcohol and began abusing all of us. Dad was a very nice dad while he did not drink. Except for times when he would lose his temper momentarily while punishing us kids. Dad was a very old-fashioned father, cutting down a switch from the tree and walloping us on the spot.

However, when Dad turned into a very mad drunk, we didn't dare be in his vicinity. Otherwise, his beatings would take on a whole new world of their own, and he would hit us with whatever was nearby (hangers, sticks, books, kitchen utensils, his belt, a work boot, pan, etc.). I remember hiding and falling asleep in my closet most nights Dad was home and drunk. Thankfully, he took to midnight work shifts often.

But never mind me and my beatings. Many times, as I grew older and came to understand what went on, I became more distraught upon hearing Mom screaming in pain. Dad would lash out at her for any reason or no reason at all. We could be simply sitting at the dinner table eating, and he would suddenly slam his full dinner plate and all on the wall next to Mother. Later on, we could hear Mom screaming and crying when he hurt her. As I got older, I got bolder and would rush out to defend our mother.

Nevertheless, I would be met with a slap or chased away by my father since he did not want me in the middle of his mess. I would try to talk with Mom after Dad beat and maimed her, but she wouldn't allow me to speak. She wanted to forget. Unfortunately, calling the police was not even thought of back then—doing so would undoubtedly exacerbate the situation and end up with my mother getting more beatings. Since Mom was not allowed to work or drive a car, she was pretty much a prisoner in her own home.

It took a lifetime of studies to come to an understanding late in my father's life that he was under a lot of pressure and had no clue how to handle things. Not to make excuses for his bad ways. He just had no help. I figured I learned a lot from that experience with my father. I learned so much that I went out of my way to treat my own family so differently. I never wanted to be abusive and had to learn on my own early how to hold the horses on great emotions that get out of hand and onto the body.

Our parents never showed any love emotions to each other or to us siblings after our first four to five years. For me, I had to learn how to trust and love once grown up and away from home, especially when it came to my first husband.

During the years of my on-again, off-again marriage to husband number one, something horrendous happened that shook up my entire family and those around me. My one and only younger sister was murdered! Yes, murdered!

There was lots more to the death of my only sister. But, alas, it would be a book in and of itself. Suffice it to say, my parents, my siblings, and I were all completely devastated and forever changed.

Then another family devastation occurred five years later, in the same month! My brother had been in an accident driving his chopper motorcycle (without his helmet)!

My dear best life friend, my dear brother, lay in a coma for seven days. My mom and I were there with him when he flatlined and then pronounced deceased. The world was caving in on us with more unbelievable horribleness. My brother's death left a gigantic hole in all our hearts. My brother's death happened in 1978, and even in 2022, I still feel the great void and miss him greatly!

My second husband was Rudy—he had health problems, quadruple bypass surgery, and aortic valve replacement in 1990. Not too long after the surgery, he developed chronic congestive heart failure, shrunk down to 116 pounds (after being 185) over the course of almost two years, and looked like a person suffering from starvation. Because he was—Starving! The advanced congestive heart failure that haunted him made him forget altogether about food.

Hospice wasn't much in the works back in the early 1990s, so Rudy spent most of his last months in the hospital. The day he died, he had me pick him up and take him home, where he had a heart attack within an hour. Paramedics rushed him to the hospital, performing CPR all the way, but he died.

A year after Rudy's death, a small pickup truck nearly killed me while I walked in a mall parking lot. The driver didn't see me and hit me hard enough to send me far into the air (as reported by a friend nearby). I suffered a broken pelvis, shattered shoulder, and many lacerations, from head to toe, since I was tossed high into the air and then down onto the pavement.

I ended up in the hospital for two weeks—One week flat on my back. Since I had so much pain, I was administered two types of pain meds. I remember people visiting me that I found out much later that they never visited. That was very disappointing! I imagined my late husband, Rudy arranging the gold thumbtacks on the bulletin board nearby into the words, "I love you."

I came home to an empty but flooded condo! My parents had driven me home and had to help me find help quickly. Thank goodness for the pain meds. Otherwise, I would have had a breakdown right then and there. That was just too much to take. I was in a wheelchair, could barely walk, and had a destroyed shoulder. And, a flooded home! What a mess!

Lucky for me, my dear son was able to get leave from the Air Force for a month and come help care for me. I felt like a complete ambulatory failure. Thankfully, the drugs dulled my senses so that I did not sit and cry continuously. Thank God for my son! He found a shower chair so that I could finally bathe! I managed that on my own, but it was challenging moving around.

Sleeping was another problem. I never liked sleeping on my back. But after my body was thrashed by the truck, I was no longer able to sleep any way BUT flat on my back. I Couldn't sleep on my good side otherwise the shattered shoulder would hang and be in excruciating pain.

I continued my extremely challenging recovery, and a year later, reconstructive surgery for my shoulder was a failure. I could no longer lift my arm high enough to brush my hair or do a lot of things. I was devastated. My husband, Rudy, had been gone two years, I was nearly killed, and I had been laid off from my job even though I had been on disability. I thought I had renewed hope of being able to use my shoulder again, but after the reconstructive surgery failure, I was devastated. Again! But that did not last long because I had to take care of myself. I knew I couldn't just feel sorry for myself. What good would that do. I had to figure it out. Get back up and tackle what needed to be done and get back to life. I planned to go back to school the following January. But then tragedy struck again.

January of 1995, during a particularly rainy first day at school, I stepped on a slippery area and took a bad fall. I experienced a badly broken ankle and was in a wheelchair for six weeks. I was told I needed surgery by the same doctor who ruined my shoulder, so, needless to say, I never had surgery and never went back to school. Instead, five years later, I began ballroom and swing dance lessons. Always determined. Never giving up!

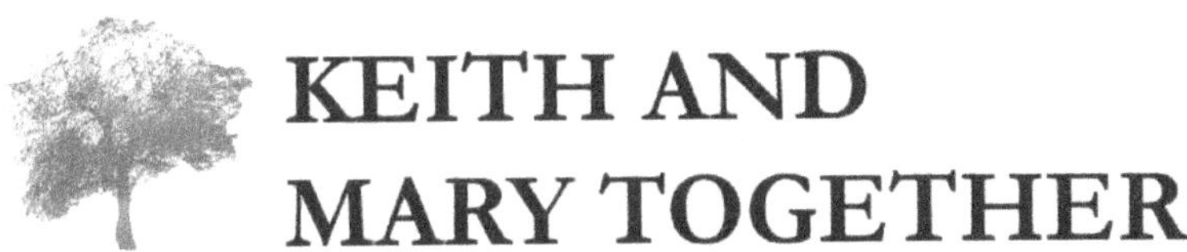# KEITH AND MARY TOGETHER

Gone Quackers

YEARS AFTER RUDY PASSED and my near-death scrape, I finally was back among the living. One day, a friend at work handed me a flyer that caught my eye. It was all about learning to dance—ballroom dance. Since one of my girlfriends had lost her husband recently, I recommended she join me in taking ballroom dance lessons. I had always loved dancing. Taking on ballroom dancing with a bum ankle plus messed up shoulder was challenging, but I persevered because I found so much joy in dancing.

After Keith's wife walked out on him, he was incredibly distraught and sought therapy for his depression. The therapist advised him to try dance lessons because where else can a man hold a woman in his arms and have the best exercise!

Keith also began to take ballroom classes with the same company I was using, a year later. Keith had never danced in his life—not even freestyle dancing. Later on, Keith told me his previous wife wanted him to dance, but he would not dance at all. I had tap and ballet dancing growing up and then freestyle dancing at the clubs in my early adult life.

Keith told me he began lessons with a lot of trepidation about doing something he had never wanted to do and feeling inept. He was also anxious about getting back out there among women.

So, chance or kismet or alignment with the stars led us to meet in the middle of the year 2002. Or was it Keith's grandmother's doing? Or was it the universe and God's plan? Perhaps some of everything!

With much joy abounding, Keith and I met in 2002 while taking ballroom dance classes. The dance teacher directed us to change partners—all women moved to the partner on the right—I moved but kept my eyes on the instructor, who was instructing and talking at the time. As I offered my hands to my next partner, I heard a loud duck "quacking" noise near me and jerked my head up quickly to see my current partner, who held me in his arms. I smiled and said, "hello." The guy holding my hands and body was "quacking" "Hello" back to me. I thought, well, now, he is a funny guy quacking like Donald Duck to me. Was that his hello? Hmmm?

That is the first time I remember Keith. The dance classes were held all over the South Bay at various venues. I remembered him first at the Temple Hall in Torrance. Keith told the story that he remembered me first at the famous Mayflower Ballroom in Inglewood. Later, we would find out that his grandmother used to dance at that Mayflower Ballroom, where she met her husband back in the 1950s. It was always the talk that Keith's grandmother helped get us together. The spirits moved us in a dancing way!

After we first caught each other's gaze, we continued to run into each other at various dance venues for lessons, dance parties, or practice. The turning point in our relationship came at the end of one West Coast Swing class. I stood catching my breath after a good workout and talking to Keith. I mentioned I was parched and needed to get home to get a drink. Keith followed that and told me that he had a cold drink for me at his place, which was nearby. He also mentioned that he had to get home to feed his foreign exchange students.

That made me more at ease about going to his home. It wasn't like me to follow men home. So, I followed him a short distance to his lovely home. After the French and Japanese students left the table to study Spanish together, Keith and I ended up chatting for hours. It was easy to talk with Keith, and I felt that we became hard and fast friends that night.

We began to contact each other to coordinate our meetings at classes and dances. We always sat with and danced together and talked a lot. I didn't have any romantic thoughts of Keith at the time. I thought that we each needed a friend, and that's what we were— friends. Our friendship blossomed over time. I thought we fit perfectly as a dance couple since both of us were on the short side of stature. I had another year of dance experience over Keith's experience (as well as a lifetime of other dancing), so I enjoyed helping him learn new steps.

One night as we walked to the parking lot after a dance lesson, we stopped for a quick moment, and I looked up at him and went onto my tippy toes and gave Keith a quick kiss on his mouth. Keith, taken by surprise, just stood there, not making a sound. I don't know what made me do that! Guess the dancing was more romantic that night? But I didn't aim too well when I tried to kiss him since I didn't find much of his lips. I told him goodnight and walked fast to my friends patiently waiting in their car.

We girls took turns driving our group to lessons. I was crazily laughing when I jumped inside the waiting car and quickly exclaimed that "He has no lips." I told them about trying to kiss him, but he had no lips. My girlfriends and I were all hysterically laughing the whole way home. It would be a while more before I would find his natural lips!

In November of 2002, I got brave again and asked him to join me in attending the yearly Thanksgiving Extravaganza church service.

Keith and I always thought of the Thanksgiving Mass/Service as our first actual date.

He picked me up in his big blue truck. This would be the first time I rode in his vehicle. It was so tall off the ground that I needed help jumping up into the seat and getting down. I needed a ladder. But I don't think Keith was in a hurry to accommodate a ladder since he was obviously enjoying being the one to help me up and out of the cab in his high truck. You see, Keith was a legs man! And yes, I often wore skirts!

Keith was astounded by the church service. Hawaiians blew the conch shell at the entrance, announcing the mass beginning. They processed in with large displays of leis, which they gifted to all the priests in attendance. The Hawaiian choir sang gorgeous hymns, then the Spanish choir and Vietnamese choir took their turns and sang more songs in their native languages.

Of course, during the whole service when we had singing, I was singing my best. My voice was in good shape since I sang in the church and community choirs.

I want to think that I hooked Keith with my voice, going to a Thanksgiving Day service at my church on our first actual date. Since I was in the choir (usually on Sundays, but not that day), I knew the music well. I think I made a few believers when it came to singing the "Lord's Prayer" by Albert Malotte. I sang bel canto—operatic-like. When I sang, everyone heard. And, that day, I sang with gusto as we held hands. After the song finished, we wished each other "peace," and Keith passed the peace to me by planting a kiss on my lips. Finally, I had found his actual lips in church! Sparks were flying between us two!

Keith and I continued to see each other as often as we could. That was about the time when I started to pick up dinners and meet Keith at his mother's care center so we could visit with her while we ate our dinner before going off to dance classes. By then, we attended up to four dance classes during the week and sometimes another class on the weekends. Immerse yourself, and practice is what they recommended in learning to dance, and we did.

Things heated up and got more serious as the following year moved along. At first, I still considered him a friend, then a good friend, and even a best friend; then, I realized I was falling in love with him. Finally, I knew that I loved Keith. By then, it had been eleven years since I had kissed the dead lips of Rudy. After I found Keith's living lips, or let's say he found my lips, Keith had reignited my spirit once again, and I was alive and happy! We were delighted. More extensive sparks were flying!

It was tricky for Keith to proclaim his love for me. I felt it in his actions and care toward me. But, because of the hurt that Keith experienced in his past, it would be a while before he would fully commit to Love. Finally, in the spring of 2003, he exclaimed with teary eyes that he loved me, and it was a joyous time for both of us.

I was ecstatic that I had found a lifelong companion with a great zest for life, straightforward, upright, truth-bearing, and, best of all, a most playful partner. Once a kid, always a kid (as we would say to each other).

Keith Proposed

WE BELONGED TO THE AREA dance club that met twice a month at a local hall for dance lessons and social practice. The club had an ongoing newsletter that put out a request for stories on how couples had met. Of course, I had to write about our story, so I entered our account for consideration. After the dance class, there was always a break with announcements. It was no different that evening, except the club president called Keith up to talk about the story I wrote. I stood there dumbfounded, wondering why he was up there while I was the one that wrote the story. My hands were defiantly placed on my hips, ready to say, "Wait a minute, I wrote this." But of course, I said nothing because the next thing I knew, Keith was speaking a bit about how we first met, and then he asked me to come up. Only Keith started coming toward me and met me on the dance floor. There, before the whole crowd and me, he got down on one knee and pulled out THE RING and held it up, surprisingly asking me if I would Marry Him! I said "Yes," of course! And he placed the glimmery, shiny, brilliant engagement ring on my finger. Then suddenly came two more people in our direction, one with flowers in hand and the other holding a cake. They cut the cake and handed me the flowers. It was a great evening, which I will never forget for as long as I live.

2003 Fairy-Tale Wedding

WE CHOSE TO BE MARRIED in November of the same year, and no, we didn't wait. We were not young anymore, and there was no reason to wait. Since both of us had been married before, we wanted to get a head start of doing it right, so, long before the wedding, we started with weekly counseling with a couple's therapist who used God and his love for us in her therapy.

We found that we made a good solid fit as a couple since we both had lived through some really tough times already in our lives. We figured those hard epochs had to build our strengths and resolve. As life evolved, we would find out just how much fortitude our union contained years later.

Later on, to solidify that we were headed in the right direction, a priest would tell us we needed no interview with him before the wedding because our marriage, per the priest, was already made in heaven. It was like magic because every obstacle melted away effortlessly.

Keith had been married twice before but never in the Catholic church. Both marriages needed annulments in the eyes of the church. They both turned out to be easier done than expected. My previous marriages were also not with the church, and I had previously taken care of everything when I joined the Catholic church, so I was ready.

Everything seamlessly fell into place neatly. November, everyone would ask; why get married in November? There is a reason for this. First, we gave the month some positive vibes, feelings, and thoughts.

You see, for the longest time, November had been a sad month because two of my siblings and my father ALL passed away in November. So, Keith and I chose November to interject some happy times and thoughts. Plus, we wanted to thank God for helping us find each other by getting married the nearest day we could to Thanksgiving.

We married the Saturday after Thanksgiving. It was the storybook church wedding we both had been dreaming about all our lives. Keith, as my handsome, proud man standing up there beaming with love, all dressed to the nines and welcoming me and joining with God. Happy, teary-eyed friends watched as the eight-foot-long train and equally long bridal veil trailed behind me. We made our union the strongest ever and absolutely unbreakable. Our first dance and lifetime couple motto was always "Now and Forever."

Keith and I met dancing, and we continued to dance for as long as life would allow us to be together. Often, we searched for dances and balls to attend to hone our skills. We loved dancing so much that we took dance lessons of all types as often as possible. We loved New Year's Eve. We dressed to the "nines" and champagned, ate, and danced until we could barely walk, and then we danced again. Yes, we danced each year into the next.

Of course, as all our friends knew, our ultimate objective every year was to be present at the famed vintage Avalon Ball on Santa Catalina Island. Live music in the grand, humungous circular ballroom like they had in the roaring twenties and thirties.

Keith and I loved to dress up as people did in the 1920s and 1930s and pretend. It was our yearly strut to the ball that we looked forward to each year. After getting all dolled up and having photos taken by hotel staff or each other, we would begin our walk to the ball from the hotel.

We had to go early enough to saunter, pausing for photos along the way and being first in line. Our strut down the lane would entail our walk through the arched entryway to the walkway along the ocean and the port. People would walk past us in both directions, with most people commenting on how well we looked, asking for photos, and offering to take our pictures with our equipment.

We put many smiles on folks' faces each and every year. One year our image appeared in the Islander newspaper for the city of Avalon. We danced about sixteen Avalon Balls in our nearly seventeen years of marriage. I have to think that the Avalon Ball for 2020 canceled because of Keith's demise. But reality says it was because of the COVID-19 virus.

"When you dance, your purpose is not to get to a certain place on the floor. It's to enjoy each step along the way." (Dr. Wayne Dyer)

Our Convictions

SINCE KEITH AND I ALWAYS placed God at the core of our being, our story must include material about our religious convictions individually as well as our faith as a couple. Somewhere in the midst of our many talks at the forefront of our friendship, Keith spoke to me about his parents baptizing him and raising him Catholic. His parents guided him and helped him achieve all the steps needed to gain his full confirmation by his teen years. That meant he was a full-fledged Catholic.

Raised Catholic, I was puzzled why Keith's two previous marriages had not been with the Catholic church. But Keith reminded me that back then, both parties had to be Catholic to be married in a Catholic church. And, since it was such an ordeal converting to another religion, it was easier to get married elsewhere.

After his second wife dumped him, Keith took solace from a priest at a local church. He still considered himself a Catholic. The priest took no pity on him, even though Keith's wife had left him. The priest told Keith in order to continue going to the Catholic church, the Catholic church would require Keith to make amends with his wife and rejoin with her in their marriage.

Keith was greatly offended by the priest and the church and turned away from the Catholic religion entirely. Meanwhile, he found a small, comforting church to attend. When I met Keith and found he was attending a Foursquare church, I was interested in learning more and accompanied Keith to the church services on Saturday and Wednesday nights. At the same time, I kept up with my services at my neighborhood Catholic church on Sundays.

I really got to know Keith while attending church services with him. It is profoundly enriching witnessing a man in his religious time with God. The pastor of the Foursquare church incredibly moved me. The pastor was feeding our souls! But the Catholic church was not finished with Keith.

While we got Keith ready for marriage in the Catholic church by getting his previous marriages annulled, we met up with one of the most outstanding Irish priests of all time. He told Keith just what Keith needed to hear. He apologized on behalf of the Catholic church for sending him away in his time of need (after his wife left him) and offered amends and renewed ways with the Catholic church should he want to come back.

Once again, Keith would hear apologies when we attended a required pre-wedding seminar. The attending priest at the conference echoed the great Irish priest in apologizing greatly. The Catholic church had turned a corner by letting its people know that they could come to the Catholic church even if they were divorced. And they could remarry in the Catholic church. "Me Paenitet," the priest said. Which is "I'm sorry" in Latin.

Since it was getting hectic for us to go to so many church services, we finally decided that we would only go to the Catholic church where we both wanted to get married. We had finally found the perfect place for both of our souls.

THE CANCER JOURNEY BEGAN–EARLY 2009

During most of the eleven years of his cancer journey, Keith journaled about his experiences. For the most part, I chronicled Keith's writings in this cancer journey story. As I have written earlier, Keith expressed his wishes often that he wanted very much to pass along his experiences to help others. Being key to this writing, Keith and I prayerfully ask you to join us in reading this cancer account. Come along as you might find something that Keith (or we) experienced to help you or your loved one(s) fight for their life. I might add that recently, in 2022, I have had several friends and friends of friends contact me for information to help them deal with their cancer. I've got to tell you that it was most satisfying to be helpful to them. I knew Keith loved that what he went through helped others. Don't miss Keith's last entry at the end.

Along with the cancer journey writings are chapters with immense information about the different complementary methods (complimentary to the medical methods) that assisted Keith to thrive throughout his cancer journey.

Keith's story began with his first entry in his journal that he kept on his laptop computer. I have italicized Keith's journal writings for the remainder of the book.

This story started on February 2, 2009, at a dance class when I was stricken with an intestinal pain that made me double over and was so strong that I felt like I would pass out. I sat for about half an hour and was able to drive home, at which time I had my wife go to the store for a laxative to relieve the big gas bubble within my intestine.

After a few hours, the gas bubble escaped, and the pain went away, which put me back into normal mode. I kept up the laxative for five days and was very fine. Then, on February 16, 2009, I had another attack. I restarted the laxative and made an appointment with a doctor to see what was up.

The doctor saw me on February 25, 2009, and told me to do an enema and take MiraLAX for seven days to clean everything out, but if I was to begin throwing up, I needed to go to the hospital for films of my intestines.

During this time, I was fine in the morning when I got up, but I became more and more distressed as the day progressed. I had like a volcano going off in my intestines. The gas was coming back through the intestines to my stomach. Then every night in bed, I would pass the gas, and I was fine in the morning.

Finally, on March 4, 2009, I got up and started to throw up bile and decided to go to the emergency room at the hospital. I spent all day and most of the night in the emergency room. About nine p.m., I was admitted to the hospital for an operation on March 5, 2009. I was told that I had a complete blockage in my colon, and it needed to come out.

For me, Keith's wife, this experience was so unbelievable. Keith had been "Mr. Healthy," always taking huge, healthy salads with him for lunch five days a week. At work, Keith walked stairs everywhere, daily, at the high-rise building where he was chief engineer. And, we danced a great deal. Obviously, he was in great shape. So, it made no sense that this horrible malady would befall Keith.

Emergency Surgery

IT WAS INCREDIBLY HEARTBREAKING to see Keith in so much agonizing pain. But amid the pain, he was making funnies during the time he spent in the ER room. During one of his humorous times, I had stepped away from his room for a bit, and when I returned, he told me that a young lady, very short of stature, had appeared and said to him that they had a date for the next day. Keith asked the newly met surgeon if she had told his wife (me) about their date? Of course, anyone in hearing distance laughed it up. Laughing it up is how Keith dealt with so much in life. Laughter was the best medicine—Giggling certainly helped during tense times.

Before the surgery, I remember wanting to grab Keith with my whole being and hug him tight, but I could only hug Keith halfway since he was lying on a gurney (waiting to go to surgery). We kissed and, of course, told each other we loved the other a few times to be sure the other heard it and knew we meant it with both hearts. We always made sure to tell each other we loved each other whenever we departed to go anywhere, and this was a big, scary thing to say our "I Love Yous," not knowing if we would ever see each other again. I was able to be with him until they wheeled him into the elevator to take him down to the surgery area. Then I sat myself down in the large waiting room full of stiff, staunch sofas and chairs. I tried to read the magazines located on the table near me, but instead, I just sat there numb with worry.

It's Cancer!

AS I RECALL, I did not have a smartphone back in 2009, just a flip phone, so there was no surfing the internet, checking Facebook, Instagram, or emails back then. I worried as my eyes watched the big hospital clock on the wall next to the door. The hours drifted slowly.

I thought it was way past the slated finish time of the surgery, and I was plenty worried. Why was it taking so long? I kept my eyes trained on the door that all doctors came through to talk with families. Finally, the surgeon came through the door, and our eyes locked immediately. She didn't hurry to me but took her time. She wore a serious face, and no doubt had something to tell me. I was surprised when she sat on the sofa next to me. After all, this was a very crowded waiting room full of people. She didn't talk loudly, but I didn't care. I carefully listened and focused on her. She was not smiling. She told me it took a while to get going on the surgery. Someone was late or something. I said in my head, "Get going; tell me about Keith."

Alarmed and frightened by the words, Keith's surgeon spoke to me, "Cancer *WAS* found in the colon, lymph nodes, and on the liver." I sat glued to the uncomfortable, large waiting room sofa with the doctor next to me. My face tickled with the dripping tears, but I paid little attention since I concentrated hard on what the doctor told me. Nothing else mattered. Not even the people whispering the word "cancer" around us mattered.

Then she told me that she opened Keith up, and yes, she resected his colon. She found cancer there in the obstruction and surrounding lymph nodes, as well as two lesions on the outside of the liver. She relayed that she removed all the cancer she could see. She told me she would recommend an oncologist to see Keith and plan a course of action. I asked her, "Are you sure it's cancer?" She replied, "Sorry, yes, it is cancer. I've operated for many years and know what cancer looks like, and this is cancer. Sorry again." At that point, tears were pouring down my face. But I hardly noticed them and gently pushed them out of my view with my fingers.

The surgeon went on to tell me that Keith would be in recovery for an hour and then moved to a hospital room, and then I would be allowed to see him. Then she left me there sitting on the sofa with an entire room of people surrounding me but left me feeling completely alone with the thoughts she had expended upon me. After the doctor left me, I realized the tears and rushed off to find tissues and headed directly to the hospital chapel. Before entering the chapel, I stopped just outside and scribbled a request in the prayer book for Keith (while tears still flowed).

Entering the chapel, I found a cushioned seat and pulled the kneeler down. Thankful no one was there, beseeching prayers emanated from me in a fervent voice. "Please, God, I beg for the life of my blessed husband. Please, OH Dear God, please spare Keith's life and rid his body of the evil cancer and revive him back to happiness." I didn't stop there. I also prayed and requested intercession by the saints for their most gracious help.

Then, I prayed and asked for the intercession of our Blessed Mother, Mary. As I prayed and requested her help, I felt overwhelmed but also consoled. Perhaps I felt her loving arms surround and hug me. I sobbed as I prayed, with heavy tears bursting forth from my senses and pouring onto the tiled floor below. As we come to know, my prayers then, and our many prayers since, would repeatedly help Keith during the next eleven years.

I wept as I recalled and wrote this story. My heavily flowing tears kept coming as I remembered and played that memory, over and over, in my mind. The memory was as evident as the day it happened.

After Keith came home from the hospital the first time, he started writing a journal. Here in Keith's own words, you get a feel for how he thought of the news of Cancer and the ordeal he had just lived.

At noon I went into surgery and was back in my room at four p.m. The next day on March 6, 2009, a doctor whom I had never seen before came into my room and informed me that the blockage within my colon was cancer. This doctor went on to say that the fatty tissue next to the colon wall was removed, nine lymph nodes were found to be cancerous, and two spots on my liver were biopsied and found to be cancer. At this point, he told me that I was a stage 4 cancer patient and the usual prognosis was a few months but he wanted to get me started on Chemo as soon as possible to give me more time, hopefully.

How did I feel? Well, at first, I thought someone was playing a joke on me. How could I feel so good and then have this in less than two weeks? After I got over the shock, I still felt that this was not happening and that it was all a mistake.

Before I went out and told everyone that it had to be a mistake, I wanted to be pain-free and out of the hospital. I also found a bag hanging from my abdomen area that was attached to what was left of my colon; I was told it was a colostomy. What the hell is a colostomy?

Well, as I soon found out, this was to be my only way of going to the restroom. I no longer used my butt, and it all came out into this bag. Now I felt like a dog with a pooper scooper attached to my skin.

My nurses were so concerned about this bag that they kept checking it every time they came into my room. I was not passing anything, no gas, no solids, no liquids, nothing. I started asking everyone when does this come off, and I go back to being a human and not a dog!

The answer I received was maybe in a year or maybe never. Okay, so now I knew that all this was a joke and a horrible joke at that. Wow!! I went in for surgery and came out with Cancer and a colostomy all in one day at the hospital.

Well, the weekend came and went, and my surgeon (a very young-looking lady) came in on Monday. She confirmed that this was not a joke but was really happening and that now my intestines were paralyzed and that I would not have food until the bag started passing gas and my gut started making noise.

There I was in the hospital with a bag on my side, a very large scar on my abdomen and chest, a doctor talking about chemo, no food or water until my bag started to get stuff in it. I also noticed that I had this tube stuck in my nose and went all the way into my stomach. I asked the Doc when is this thing coming out? Again, I received the answer of not until your bag starts doing something.

The days turned into weeks, and after two weeks, I started seeing things happen in the bag. Wow! The tube came out and, they started giving me water and lots of liquids for food. After a day of that, I started throwing up again, and in the middle of the night, they came in and forced that tube back into my nose and down into my stomach.

They kept telling me to swallow that tube, and I just kept throwing it up, so in came this expert nurse, and she had me eat ice chips to get the tube started, and it worked. Down it went! I do not recommend putting a nasogastric tube in your nose down to your stomach. Now, another few days went by, and they decided to take out this tube again and put me back on the liquid diet.

This time I get past the liquid and down to real food. The hospital released me, and I got to go home. At home, I eat, and guess what? I threw up again, and I ended up back in the emergency room with my surgeon asking me what happened? She puts that tube back into my nose, and I am put in a room again with no food and no water.

Another week goes by, and they tell me that I need to eat, so they put me on a PICC line with intravenous food. This liquid sugar water meant that I had to have my sugar tested every hour—what a pain in the fingers.

Okay, what in the world is a PICC line? A PICC line is a small tube that they put inside a large vein in your arm, and it goes all the way to your heart, where the liquid is pumped throughout your body without destroying your veins.

A week or so later, the surgeon came in and told me that she had been praying for me and that something was wrong. My intestines should be working after all this time, so she wanted to go back and cut into me and see what was wrong.

But first, she sends me to X-Ray for a few shots so she can pick out the best place to cut in. I get into X-Ray, and the tech gives me contrast to drink (Two Quart Bottles). I told her that I couldn't drink or eat anything. Well, she put the contrast into a very big syringe and proceeded to pump it through my nose tube right into my stomach.

This is another one of those things that I DO NOT RECOMMEND! After all, that contrast makes it into my stomach; they wait about ten minutes and start taking pictures (x-rays). First, it was with x-rays of me lying flat on my back. Then, on my side, on the other side, then standing up front and back.

All of a sudden, I see this bag that is hanging on my side is full, and it is really getting big (ballooning). The technician sees it also and puts me in the restroom to empty it. After I emptied the bag, it was back to the pictures.

However, before they can set up for the next series, the bag fills up again. I ended up emptying three bags before the x-rays finished. I finally got back to my room, and the surgeon came in and was very happy with the three full bags and, she says, out comes the tube and back on liquids.

After that, I was given soft foods and finally, after three days, real food. My system was now working, I was able to go home, and I stayed home this time.

Before I left the hospital, they took out my PICC line and put in a port-a-cath, which is another type of PICC line. This little device sits under your skin, just under your neck, in your chest, and has a tube that goes into your jugular vein.

The port-a-cath is for chemotherapy infusions. I was to start chemotherapy a week after the insertion, which was around the 20th of April (about six weeks after surgery). Here is where a difference of opinions from doctor to doctor drives a person crazy.

The port-a-cath doctor stated that I should wait for at least a week before using the device because of infection. I did not want to go back into the hospital with an infection, so I made the decision to tell the chemo doctor I needed to wait a week as per the port-a-cath doctor's advice. It was my first experience being the leader of my own treatments and cure.

The chemo nurse told me that I was being very silly, that she had given chemo on the same day as the install of a port-a-cath before with no problems. I just told her not with me, and we waited the week. One week later, I was sitting in chemo and getting my first dose of chemo.

Chemo is a group of drugs that, when put all together, kills cancer along with every other healthy cell in your body. I like to call it poison to the body, so why do we do it? To try to get back to our regular lives (which will never be the same again) and start living life again. The chemo nurse listed all the side effects that I would suffer (which were many), and in my mind, I thought I was stronger than these other persons, and I could do this better than other persons in the world.

Chemo is everything you have ever heard about, but the experience is worse than they tell you because it is happening to you. After my first chemo, I had more side effects than the nurse told me. I had numb fingers, toes, mouth, and throat. I could not touch anything cold or drink anything cold without having my throat close up, or my hands get stuck in one position after picking up something cold.

I know that people wore gloves to walk in the snow but get a drink out of the refrigerator? Well, I was then wearing big thick gloves just to reach into the fridge and forget the freezer. The significant side effect I had that I was not told about was the pain (significant pain) in my mouth and neck whenever I took my first bite of food. It would put you on the floor.

It was so bad, and then the second bite, there was nothing. I mean, not even an ouch was felt on the second bite (very strange effect). The side effects lasted about four days the first time, and things went back to normal. One week after my first chemo treatment, my port-a-cath started to itch and itch all the time. I just figured that it was healing like most other wounds would heal.

The Sunday before my second chemo on Monday, my wife noticed that my port-a-cath area looked very red and swollen (infected). Back to the hospital emergency room to find out that the port had gotten infected after just one use.

The hospital took the port out and put me on all kinds of meds to kill the infection. I spent seven days in the hospital to kill the infection. The day I was to leave the hospital, they installed a PICC line into my left arm so my chemo could continue. Two weeks after the infected port, I was back in the infusion (chemo lounge) room with the chemo nurse, and she was very confused about the PICC line.

After going through hell the previous week and not being in good humor that day, I told her that it was 100% her fault and I would never forgive her for the pain I went through. She told me that she had been a chemo nurse for over twenty-four years and never had a port problem. After that and other bad experiences while in her care, I wonder why she still remained a chemo nurse.

Chemo went on for the next three months, one treatment every other week with one week off between each chemo treatment. During this time, I was working the weeks I did not have Chemo. I thought I could work after they took the chemo pump off of me on Wednesday, but I soon gave up that idea, it was just too hard, and I felt just so bad for the next two days.

The Oxaliplatin was just too hard on me for me to go to work on Thursday and Friday of the same week as Chemo. After the three months of Chemo (six treatments), I was taken off chemo to allow my body to rest for twelve weeks. Doctors set me up for the reconnection operation and the Ablation of the cancer tumors in my liver. They first did a PET scan, which showed that the liver's two tumors had reduced to only a shadow, and that was good news.

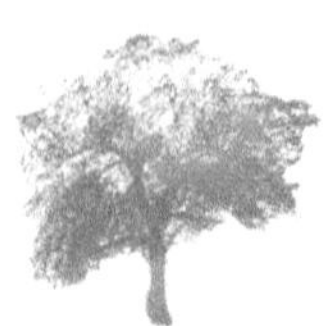

HOPE AND FAITH

"There is no profit in curing the body if, in the process, we destroy the soul." (Samuel Golter)

Hope and Faith. Much of how we both had always lived—with an abundance of Hope and a great deal of Faith. But the surgery and cancer news meant a new urgent need for both. We never lost hope, and we often called upon our faith, our religion, to take care of our souls.

As Keith rested in his sterile hospital environment, a day after his first surgery, after being advised by his new oncologist that he only had a few months to live, he turned to God for help. We both prayed eagerly for the magical comfort of God and our universe.

It would've been easy for Keith to be furious at God since he lost his father to cancer. He had already paid his dues. However, Keith did not think like that. He never got mad, nor did he blame the cancer on God or anyone, including himself. Besides, he reverently believed that God would see him through this cursed cancer jail.

A motivating quote by Dr. Wayne Dyer says, "Faith is the complete reliance on the power and goodness of spirit and the firm belief that you are always connected to this goodness." *(Faith Affirming*, www.waynedyer.com)

Keith's religious faith had always been strong. But I witnessed that his faith (and mine) grew in strength during Keith's cancer journey. Priests were often involved in preparation for his never-ending surgeries and procedures. And, our supporters supplied nonstop prayers and upright thoughts.

Being supported by our religious beliefs helped Keith (and helped me) through the sometimes-treacherous cancer road. Without our faith, it would have been a different struggle.

Our faith and religious help came just as needed sometimes. I recall when Keith received a call from his priest asking if we could go right away to a private healing service at the chapel of our town church. He told Keith that a very famous healer from the Philippines would hold a large healing service the next day, but that Saturday afternoon, he thought it would be better to get a private healing rather than in a hugely crowded church. We agreed because the church was just minutes from our home.

Once we arrived, they ushered us to a small row of seats in the tiny chapel. Each row only held room enough for two adults. The chapel was so small. We didn't know what to expect. So, we were surprised when a Catholic service started. After the final prayers, people began lining up, in the aisles, for the priest. Behind each person in line stood two others with their arms outstretched, ready to catch those in front of them. Yes, save the person as they fell backward.

Amazed at what we were witnessing, we watched as, one by one, a person would stand erect before the priest. The priest would whisper something and seem to make a forceful blowing noise (from his mouth) right onto the person's face. As he blew on the person's face, the person would fall backward, caught by the two stationed behind, lowered to the cold floor, then laid there with eyes closed for what seemed like a minute or more before the "helpers" assisted the person to rise and leave. The treated people all seemed to be in a daze as each of them left the chapel quietly. The more we watched, the more we became more nervous. What did we get ourselves into? We were closer to the back, so should we escape? Should we leave? We didn't talk, but it was as if we each knew what we were thinking. We kept looking at each other with wondering question marks seemingly propped on our foreheads.

Before we could decide and react, it was our turn. The attendants ushered Keith and me up toward the priest (they placed me standing behind the people who would catch Keith). I could hear the priest ask Keith, "What do you want healed?" And Keith answered, "The cancer!" Then, the priest forcefully blew on Keith's face, and down Keith went, falling backward into the "catcher's" arms. Apprehension and anxiousness gnawed at me. Would I go down? I wondered.

After they helped Keith to his feet, I was next. The priest queried me with, "What do you want healed?" I quickly voiced to him, "My husband's cancer." He motioned to me to close my eyes, and I felt him blow on my face. Then, surprisingly, I fell backward without a touch! I felt at peace. I was totally relaxed. I was getting overly concerned just moments before, but now, I felt wholly tranquil and at ease. It was an amazing feeling. No one pushed me down, so how did the priest blowing on my face make me fall backward gently? Keith had gotten up by then and watched while the people helped me to my feet. We walked out of the chapel slowly, holding onto each other, praying in our minds that the healing worked for Keith.

Since we both felt in a daze of sorts, we walked to the car slowly, got in, and sat quietly in the car for a long time until we were sure our wits were prepared for the short drive home.

That healing service would be our only healing service. It was a really fantastic experience, but we never got the opportunity again. Did the healing work? I would venture it did since Keith lived many years after that healing service.

Every inch of the eleven-year cancer struggle, Keith was helped by everyone's prayers and positive thoughts. Of course, we could not have done it all without the tremendous help of our prayer and thought warriors. I say "warriors" because they were there for Keith's fight for his life.

In order to communicate with our prayer and thought groups, I found it easier to build email groups and send email blasts for the prayer requests. The response to our emails was always tremendously uplifting for us to read. As I said before, without our religion and our faith, it would have been a different kind of cancer journey. Further, it certainly would have been another struggle without our prayer and thought groups.

Next was a greeting card prayer from one of our staunchest prayer warriors.

The Power of Prayer

The greatest power God gives to us

Is the power that's found in prayer,

When we share with Him our hurts and fears

With faith that He is there.

We cannot rule our lives ourselves,

Or even find a way,

But He gives us power to find His help

Each time we kneel to pray.

(author unknown)

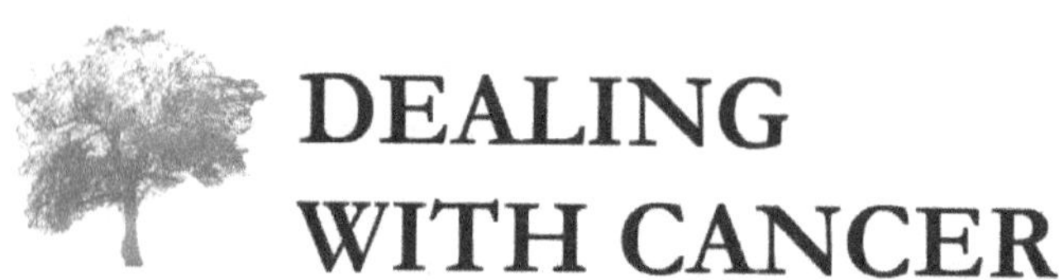

DEALING WITH CANCER

Telling All Truth

ANYONE DEALING WITH CANCER, whether as a patient or the family or friend of a cancer patient, everyone near or far from the central person deals with the psychology of the thorny subject of the scourge.

Not long ago, physicians kept the varied details of the patient's maladies close to the vest and only doled out mere crumbs. This forced the patient and others to trust the physician at their word.

With the coming of the age of information and everyone with computers and cell phones, patients and families are increasingly researching their health problems. Instead of settling, as in the past, people are demanding more details from their doctors about their cancer and how to fight the issues. Patients are also seeking second opinions and opinions of the new and unorthodox to learn of every angle of cancer riddance.

Upon learning they have cancer, patients find that their life has or soon will change dramatically as their "life turns upside down." According to Patrice Guex (1994), patients may experience great shock, be "terrified," or even "shattered."

Once the doctor announced my husband's cancer, I was the first to hear the words. I was shocked and unbelieving and waited to wake up from a nightmare. Once my husband's oncologist said the words, "You've got CANCER," Keith relayed to me that he was also experiencing the unbelieving and was also very shocked and stunned for some time.

Yes, Keith's world, our world, was topsy-turvy immediately. For the next eleven years, Keith and I were constantly readjusting to something different; something more to deal with, yet another treatment, another chemotherapy, another this or that. Each time Keith (and I) declared, "We got this!" another *New Normal* for our lives would form.

Right from the start, with the surgery to resect Keith's colon and an ostomy bag to contend with, it was a brand-new way of living for Keith. We had to learn how to care for him because suddenly he had to poop in a bag! Thankfully, this New Normal time didn't last too many months! They reconnected his colon months later, and Keith could go to the bathroom normally again. What a relief!

While fighting cancer, it is essential to continue enhancing the quality of life. To know the psychology of the mind is helpful in this process. According to Patrice Guex's book, *An Introduction to Psycho-oncology*, it is crucial to know the cancer's "psychological, psycho-social and behavioural aspects." Cancer patients strive to make sense of what they are going through. They want to know the why and the how. The patient might be suffering from much fearfulness of "alienation," "mutilation," ("change in self-image"), "loss of control," and "vulnerability." (Patrice Guex, 1994, 84)

Patients may experience apprehensions about being abandoned by their own family and friends once the doctors reveal cancer as well as at the end of life. Some family and friends feel that the cancerous patient should be left alone and not bothered. Some patients may even send mixed signals, allowing others to form a belief that they should be left alone. But the reality is the cancer patient needs total support 24/7. A cancer patient should not be left alone to fight the demon of cancer. It takes a village, as the saying goes.

Keith would not have survived eleven long years if I was not by his side every moment, supporting him. If he were living alone, he wouldn't have asked for help. I am not convinced that he would have gone to the hospital for the initial blockage or any other problems or asked for anyone's help for chemotherapy trips or aftercare.

Keith experienced this with some of his friends—abandonment. I found out from a couple that they thought he wanted his space. They thought it was like getting sick with the flu or cold, and they kept their distance. I had to play social director many times and bring friends back to Keith. People don't understand the difference between being sick and suffering from cancer. Some might fear chancing "catching" cancer, which is pure hogwash!

All concerned "fight to maintain a reasonable emotional balance." (Patrice Geux, 1994, 14). There is also the "adaptation to the disease." (Patrice Geux, 1994, 14, 21). At first, the patient, family, and friends deny the cancer. They don't understand and cannot comprehend that it IS real and exists inside their loved one's body. Using "unconscious phenomena" allows a person to figure out how to obtain resources and "strategies" to deal with the cancer they are denying and bring on acceptance. (Patrice Geux, 1994, 17)

Differential denial is "selective ignorance." Per the Urban Dictionary, 2014, this is "the practice of selectively ignoring distracting, irrelevant, or otherwise unnecessary information." Those fighting cancer find they are invariably living uncertainty regarding their lives and dealing with cancer. They constantly have to readjust and adapt to the new normal journey of living with cancer.

As I mentioned above, Keith was constantly adjusting and evolving as the cancer danced around inside his body. Keith didn't care to dance with cancer since I was his only dance partner!

According to Patrice Guex, using the psycho-social way with patients of cancer "should encourage…natural evolution…" of the "Stages" and follow the patient's wishes on how to proceed. (Patrice Guex, 1994, 22)

A service I wish Keith and I had available during Keith's long battle with cancer—a psycho-social worker/therapist environment. I found out about this type of assistance through a friend who advised me that she had done this type of job for many years when she worked for several oncology offices. As my friend spoke about how the therapy would work in conjunction with the oncologist's office's protocol, I became excited and told her, "I wish that provision would have been available for Keith!"

My friend told me a bit about how the psycho-social worker deals with the patient and family (of course, without giving me specific details because of HIPPA). At the first meeting with the patient and family, she would find out the cancer diagnosis and the stage of the patient's cancer. Knowing this pertinent information could help her therapy efforts.

Of course, as she advised me, everyone is different, and which therapy depends on what the therapist observes and hears during observational meetings. Sometimes a patient needs to talk or needs someone to talk with. They may not feel comfortable talking about hard subjects such as cancer with their family members. Sometimes the family members are the ones who become unavailable listeners and non-communicators. Occasionally it is the other way around. Faced with cancer can be very intimidating even to the strongest of human beings. As they say, it can bring you to your knees.

Cancer nearly did bring us to our knees many times, but every time we pulled our bootstraps up and synched on our positivity.

Since I had such a life where I had been trained and trained by so many trials, I knew I was ready to help Keith with his cancer journey.

You must know there were plenty of very scary moments. But, by the grace of God, he made it through those scary times, and on he went to the next cancer adventure.

I was greatly concerned after his first surgery because he lost so much weight. He was thin to start. And, when he experienced an infected port-a-cath, he lost even more weight.

Greatly concerning also was dealing with Keith's ostomy bag. Thankfully we had home nursing help. But most of the time, we were on our own. Without going into detail—It was a messy business! Thankful for the few times we could laugh about the ostomy bag as I recalled the time the bag passed gas while we stood in a busy, quiet elevator. It was all we could do to hold back our laughter until we were well clear of the elevator doors and chuckling like school kids.

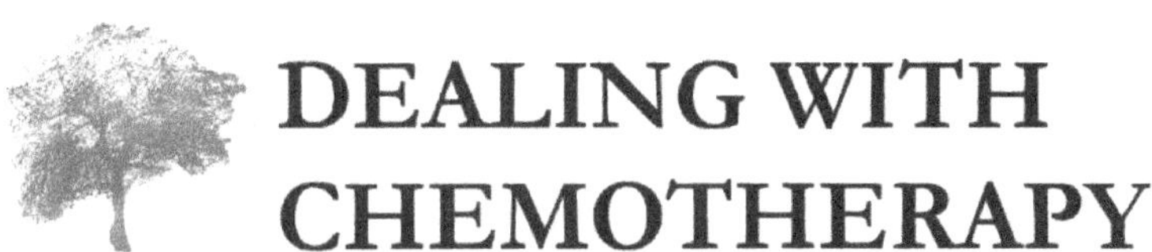 DEALING WITH CHEMOTHERAPY

Watching the pain on Keith's face as he experienced his first chemotherapy infusions and their aftereffects were hard for me to watch. But I had to watch because I cared deeply about Keith. I would not have hesitated if I could have taken on these infusions for him.

I thought Keith would faint each time he took his first bite of food. His near-fainting began after receiving his first chemotherapy infusions. At first, I had no idea what was happening and thought he was having a heart attack or something. Again (as we did often), we rushed out the paperwork, jumped on the interwebs, and read all the side effects, and yes, there on the list—jaw pain upon first bites.

Then, Keith learned the hard way, the first time he reached into the fridge for a cold drink. Cold anything went by the wayside for many months while he was on the chemotherapy drug Oxaliplatin. Thick gloves helped, but mostly I retrieved anything cold, and Keith had to let it come to room temperature to intake the product without pain. Thankfully this was in the spring and summer months. Otherwise, it would've been more painful for him in the winter.

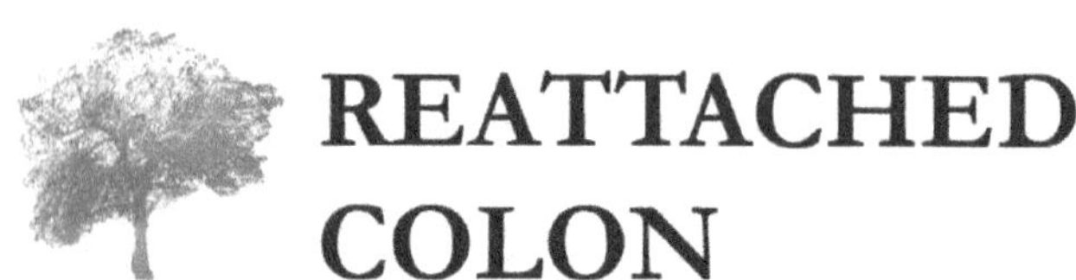# REATTACHED COLON

K eith was back at the hospital for the reattachment of his colon in August 2009. It was an exciting time because the reattachment meant losing the colostomy bag and closing the ostomy. Next, in Keith's own words, is his experience with the surgery.

I went in for the two surgeries (at the same time) on August 28, 2009, and spent about two hours on the operating table. (This is Mary: He thinks he was only in there two hours, but it was more like four to five hours) *I woke up in ICU with all kinds of tubes in me in all kinds of places.*

I guess the biggest line was in my neck, where they had what they called the C-line (central line), which meant they could feed me a pint of blood in seconds if I needed it. Why would I need it? The doctor said that when you operate on the liver, there is a possibility of a lot of blood loss all at once.

I spent three days in ICU during that time and didn't experience much pain. I had an epidural installed during the operation to keep me from having pain. Yes, the same thing women have during childbirth. Only my epidural was hooked up for the surgery and remained implanted and delivering the drug ongoing for three days and nights. Since it was an epidural near the spine, I couldn't sit up or get out of bed. I also had a pain pump, which gave me morphine every time I pushed the button or once every two hours if I did not push the button.

The morphine made me sick, and I had them remove the morphine after I left ICU. The doctors gave me some other high-end pain killer, which I did not take because I did not like how it made me feel. After some doing, I got into the First Surgical wing of the hospital in a private room. I was on no food or drink until my intestines started working again.

Gee, this sounds just like the last time I was in this hospital. After a week, they had me eating real food, and I was using my rectum again. I had to relearn bathroom skills and how to use certain muscles most people take for granted. I also found where they kept the popsicles at the nurses' station and started helping myself whenever I would go out for a walk around the ward.

When I was released, they made sure that I had a new PICC line so that the chemo could restart. Oh Goody! They told me I would need another six sessions. I restarted Chemo in September, but this time without the Oxaliplatin.

This time I was able to work on the last two days of the week and all of the next week. So, I was only off work the three days that the chemo was going into my body. At the sixth session, I figured they would pull the PICC line out, and I would be free for the rest of my life.

When the chemo nurse told me that I had only completed three sessions and not six, I was really confused. Well, a session is two weeks. So, I thought a session was only one-half of a session. The seventh chemo treatment was the worst of my life. As soon as the nurse flushed the PICC line, I knew she had done it too fast, and it curled up in my vein (in my neck), which hurt like you could not believe.

It was so horrible, and it was Christmas Eve, so I had to wait till after Christmas to have it looked at (we made an appointment at the hospital). I spent three long days in pain, and when I went in for the appointment for a look-see, they pulled the PICC line out and installed a new one in the other arm.

I then had to have the doctor who removed the coiled PICC line call the chemo nurse to instruct her that she needed to go slow when doing the PICC line's flush. Later at the next chemo (she was the only chemo nurse), again, this nurse tells me that she has been doing this work for over twenty years, and the doctors know nothing.

Well, I made sure she never flushed my PICC line fast again, and I had no more problems with the PICC line. Funny how those doctors who know nothing really helped me not have PICC line pain again. As my sessions passed from week to week, I would see the same people in the chemo room, and we would talk about everything.

One day I talked to one of the ladies receiving chemo and found out that she had the same problems that I had, and her doctor (not the same chemo doctor as mine) had told her that the tumors in her liver could not be removed. I told her that my tumors were ablated and that she should see my liver doctor.

I gave the information to her lady friend, who had taken her to chemo. While at my next chemo session, I asked about her. I found out that my liver doctor had seen her and that they were going to do the ablation on her, and that she would be a good candidate for a cure. At my last chemo session on March 3, 2010, I was able to speak to this lady, and she was so happy. She told me that I had given her a second outlook on life. I told her that GOD gave her this outlook, and all I did was give her some information that GOD had given me a few months before.

The last week in March 2010, I went in for another PET scan, and it turned out to be the best news ever. After a year's time, there was no detectable cancer anywhere in my body. WOW! I went from a stage four colon cancer to being cured in one year!! WOW, God is great! Praise the Lord and praise Jesus!

Keith wanted to celebrate, and I wanted to join in! We were joyful! We were thankful, and we wanted to share the news. Thus, we planned an elaborate dance party in April 2010, with dance lessons, food, and dancing to a live big band at our local car museum.

We even invited the doctors that operated on Keith. The first surgeon and her husband happily attended as they were interested in dancing. Everyone was happy. Keith was the happiest person. It was a long time coming, so Keith smiled ear to ear all night.

I will cherish those special times with friends, family, and doctors celebrating. Even though we would learn months later that Keith cured of cancer would be short-lived. Nevertheless, as you see, it was all about attitude—Keith's attitude, my attitude, everyone's attitude.

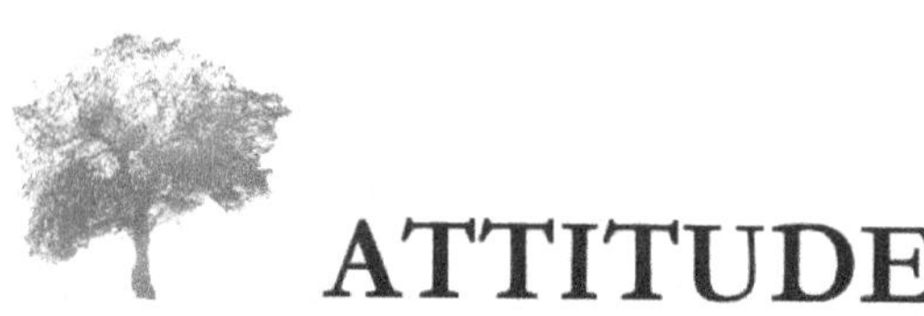

ATTITUDE

K eith, always admired for his great attributes with his everyday attitude. First and foremost were his positive thinking ways. I also considered myself a positive thinker, which helped our strong union.

There was something to be said about the Power of Positive Thinking, especially since it has been in use since ancient times by the big thinkers. For this conversation, though, I noted that for over one hundred years, the power of positive thinking had been the focus for many who wished to improve their lives. As history shows, it came to the consciousness of the people by way of the coming of the New Thought Movement of the nineteenth century.

One might think I errored in typing nineteenth century, believing positive thinking as the here and now. But in reality, the consciousness of the Power of Positive Thinking did indeed develop its roots back in the nineteenth century. Yes, back in the 1890s–1920s, there came the New Thought Movement phenomenon, where it reasoned that "sickness originates in the mind, and "right thinking" has a healing effect," according to Wikipedia. Read more via the link listed in the Glossary under New Thought Movement.

Wikipedia defines positive thinking as: "Optimism, mental attitude, interpreting everything as being best, American movement of 19th Century asserting the power of positive thinking." As we can see, positive thinking was part of the New Thought phenomenon.

The positive thinking modus operandi continued through the years with Napoleon Hill's famous quote, "If we can believe it, we can achieve it!" (Paraphrased from Hill's 1937 book, *Think and Grow Rich*)

Keith knew about the "believe it, achieve it" theory and used it often, visualizing the body rid of the cancer. From the start of Keith's journey, Keith believed that there was no cancer—that it was all a mistake by the doctors. He took action as required by the physicians, but he also kept envisioning the body clear of cancer. He kept the positive thoughts flowing constantly.

There again, positive thinking was also popularized by Norman Vincent Peale in his book *The Power of Positive Thinking*, published in 1952. Mr. Peale was considered the "father of positive thinking."

Peale's primary phrase was "Believe in yourself!" He referenced scripture to back up his book offerings with "I can do all things through Christ which strengthens me." Philippians 4:13. He also wrote, "Change your thoughts, and you change your world." Furthermore, he wrote, "You can have peace of mind, improved health, and a never-ceasing flow of energy."

Research abounds showing positive thinking has the possibility of producing and adding worth to a person's life. It's not just about delivering a good attitude. It is all about making a change.

One of Buddha's aphorisms was this astute declaration: "Every Man and Woman is the architect of their own healing and their own destiny." Wayne Dyer wrote the book *The Power of Intention* and mentioned this title as the background to the famous "The Secret." Using techniques from Buddha and Dyer can lead one to envision and create healing in their body. Since I utilized techniques from "The Secret" for over twenty-five years, long before the book and videos came out, I introduced Keith to these concepts early in our marriage. I know he used the concepts often, even before he became sick with cancer. Keith would often come to me after opening the daily mail and present a check received. He would then announce that the "The Secret" was at work. He always thought of money coming in the mail, never about bills. Half the time, he/we received money from places that we least expected.

I personally have used the concepts for "The Secret" and "The Power of Intention" and have seen them work for me, and I urged Keith to also use the techniques for healing his body.

Years before I met Keith, I felt I was in a good place. I was single and happy. But I wondered about getting older and remaining alone. So, I began my new intention thoughts and prayers. I would think of this intention and pray about it often. Usually at weekly church services but also at night before going to sleep. From my previous life experiences, I learned that one has to be very specific about prayers and thoughts. Otherwise, life can play a joke on you if you are not very specific. My thoughts and prayers were for God and the universe to find me a life companion, a husband, a short man my age, intelligent, good-looking, funny, lover of music, dancer, and Catholic. Tall order. And, I never gave up on these thoughts and prayers. I did this daily process for maybe three and a half years until one day, I attended a dance lesson class and met my future husband. However, I didn't recognize my answered prayers for some time. Nonetheless, once I realized that every single one of those items on my list was all enveloped in my dear Keith, I jumped with joy and declared, "Setting my intentions and The Secret" worked. Again!

"Surrender to a new consciousness: I can do this thing in this moment. I will receive the help I need as long as I stay with this intention and go within for assistance." (Dr. Wayne Dyer, *You Are What You Think*)

The Secret is a book, and there are some videos that explain it well. It's simply the law of attraction—Whatever you are thinking will happen. Emerges from your leading thoughts. (*The Secret*, Rhonda Byrne). Per Rhonda Byrne (The Secret, *The Greatest Secret and The Secret to Health Masterclass*), over time, we train our subconscious mind, and what we think roots in the subconscious mind. If we reprogram our subconscious minds, we can change our lives and, most notably, our health.

As everyone knows or should learn, energy makes up our body. Thus, our thoughts are made up of energy. Thoughts can cause happenings. (*Secret to Health Masterclass*, Rhonda Byrne) Therefore, if your sole focus is on the illness, then the sickness will prevail. Think more about the healing and healing will occur. Per Rhonda Byrne, thinking one thing over and over can make it happen because we are leading our subconscious.

Visualization and affirmations are mainstays within the workings of the Law of Attraction. According to Gregg Braden with the Heart Math Institute, creating a vision in your mind and focusing on believing the vision can create reality. Check out the link in the glossary under Heart Math.

Keith used visualization, along with his thoughts, to assist in his long-lasting cancer journey. He would share with me how he would envision a clean, pure white light entering through the top of his head and how the light moved slowly throughout his body, one area after another. He envisioned the white light clearing out all cancer and disease and ridding the body down through the bottoms of his feet.

Other ways to visualize were with photos of yourself when you were happiest, in the happiest setting, and the best of health. Place it where you see it every day and focus and visualize yourself in the best of health, all cancer cleared, all disease removed and gone for good. Think only of good health and refuse negativity.

As Dr. Robert H. Schuller would say during his televised shows, "Inch by inch, everything is a cinch." In 1983, he wrote a book that said it best: *Tough Times Never Last, But Tough People Do*. He inspired people with his positive thinking talk on radio, TV, and books for over fifty years. His weekly broadcasts on television and radio helped many people overcome their problems. Schuller's famous *Tough Times* book became one of Keith's mottos as well. Keith was one tough hombre.

Of course, we must mention Tony Robbins, the inspirational speaker of motivational seminars and books beginning in the 1980s. He taught and continues to teach ways to use the power of positive thinking. He says, "You can adopt this mindset and experience all the benefits of positive thinking in your own life."

All this talk about positive thinking. You probably wonder how negative thoughts or negative thinking figures into the positive-thinking ways? Why not negative thoughts? Because if a person is concentrating solely on continuous negative thinking, this narrows the thinking and focus and limits the options. Usually, negative thoughts involve fear, anger, or stress, which causes the body to go into an automatic response mode that triggers the fight-or-flight survival instinct ingrained from ancient times into our minds and body.

However, if you should be pressed by fear, anger, or stress, choosing the correct reaction using the power of positive thinking will open more avenues of response and the ability to survive the trial. Should only negative thoughts crowd your mind to a narrow focus with negative emotions and negative thinking, it will keep the mind from seeing all the other options open to handle the negative thoughts in a better, more efficient way to turn things positively.

It is recommended to learn the triggers and deal with them with thoughts of positivity to fight the negative activates. The use of a sense of humor is also beneficial. Humor is undoubtedly a positive thought process, bringing laughter to everyone.

Keith was a master at provoking laughter and dispelling negativity. He was forever "quacking" it up, especially in tight, stressful times. Keith would be quacking like Donald Duck, saying not just words but entire sentences. Along with his "quacking it up," he was the one who was quick with the dry wit. Quiet Keith would often catch people by surprise, and people either got it or did not get it. He figured those who did not get the punchline did not have a sense of humor. Keith certainly did. Keith and I knew that laughter was better than crying at any time. We tried to interject funny thoughts or ways as much as possible.

One of the most important ways of using positive thinking is giving to others. Giving to others, whether by gifting, making things for others, helping others with their lives, or just plain bringing joy to others in all ways, has a way of bringing positivity to all involved in a long-lasting way.

My precious husband, Keith, was always giving to others. There were a few doctors at his oncology office. Since he had been going through chemotherapy for so long, he knew a lot about the different therapies he had experienced and how to deal with the side effects. The doctors would often make sure new clients sat in the chemotherapy lounge chair next to Keith's chair. Usually, when a person walked into this large, linoleum-floored room with the circle of brown, plumply upholstered, comfy lounge chairs, they would witness the multitude lying back, covered with soft, cushioning, comforting blankets. Most of the time, patients filled the infusing room. Most people would have their eyes closed and possibly be sleeping to escape the effects of the chemotherapy treatment they were enduring.

Once a doctor introduced Keith to a new client, he would chat with the person and find out which chemicals they would be receiving. Then, he would try to set them at ease with information and let them know what to look out for and how to handle the different side effects, should they happen. Since most newbies had no one helping them, they were always thankful to Keith for his gracious and generous help (even if Keith himself was feeling poorly from the infusion process). Keith sure wished someone had been there to help him figure out things initially. That is the reason he always tried serving others. At the beginning of his cancer journey, Keith had no help. Before Keith started his first chemotherapy, the doctor handed a paper to him about the chemotherapy that included a list of side effects long enough to scare anyone. But no one to talk to about what to expect.

Consequently, that led Keith to support anyone going through the cancer-fighting process. Every time Keith spoke to a person in the chemotherapy lounge, the other chemo-laden persons would open their eyes and seem to be listening to Keith's message. Some of the eye-openers would speak up and ask their own questions. Clearly, there was a great need for more information about everyone's cancers and chemotherapy treatments. Keith made many friends while receiving his chemotherapy infusions and he brought smiles to those heavy laden with chemotherapy labor. Again, with a quote from Tony Robbins from his seminars and books, "The secret of living is giving." Yes, indeed, Keith was the giver!

I can hear you say just about now, but is there a scientific side of positive thinking? According to John Hopkins Medicine (JohnHopkins.org), living with positive thinking allows hope, keeps away inflammation problems, and assists in better health. "Studies also find that negative emotions can weaken immune response." "…definitely a strong link between positivity and health."

Per The Mayo Clinic online (mayoclinic.org), people see positive thinking as "you think the best is going to happen, not the worst."

Using positive thinking is an excellent way to reduce stress. Since stress is known as causing inflammation in the body and, subsequently, causing disease, remove negative thoughts, reduce stress, and have a healthier psychological mindset.

Now, courtesy of UCLA (exploreim.ucla.edu), the following is a profound statement: "Psychoneuroimmunology is an interdisciplinary field of how our thoughts and feelings influence our brain and nervous system, which temper the body's disease-fighting mechanisms." Further, they found that optimists are better fit physically and have better "immune responses."

There exists even more info about the scientific medical exploration of positive thinking. For example, the American Psychological Association promotes the "immune-brain loop" and affirms that the "brain communicates our thoughts and emotions with the body's systems, vice versa."

"Communication between the brain and immune system occurs via two major pathways—one of which is the hypothalamic-pituitary-adrenal axis (HPA axis), the body's primary stress management system. The HPA axis allows us to respond to physical and mental challenges by stimulating activity in immune cells such as T cells and natural killer cells (NK cells), regulated by cytokine messenger molecules such as interleukin-6 (IL-6)." Check out the link to more information in the Glossary under UCLA.

The power of positive thinking and an excellent "Can Do IT" attitude is what helped Keith live his eleven years with cancer. He constantly changed his thoughts to adapt and learn the "new normal" life that included cancer. And Keith did all this with much enthusiasm for life. For life is what he wanted to continue to achieve.

Be thankful. "An attitude of gratitude brings great things." — Yogi Bhajan

Keith Heals Himself

OF COURSE, AS PART OF HIS ATTITUDE, Keith wanted to heal himself. He was always reading and educating himself. He religiously made a point every morning after breakfast to sit quietly (as much as possible with his jabbering wife talking way too much (that would be me)) and read his daily portions of the *Give Us This Day* booklet. Then, move to one of his latest self-help books, such as Louise L. Hay's *You Can Heal Your Life*. (2005)

As I picked up Keith's copy of Hay's large paperback-sized book, I noticed that Keith had marked many pages by writing in the book, tagging the pages with Post-it stickies, and placing markers of papers and cards of various items in between pages. Since he had gotten this book long ago, I would assume he had read through it, but perhaps he would come back to it periodically to these specific pages? I wish I could ask him right now.

As I peruse the eloquent words of Hay's book, I do see that she recommends reading through the book and then rereading it slowly a second time. Perhaps Keith was doing just that. I can't help but notice how Keith had marked certain areas in the book. These must have resonated with him.

Keith had these denoted with his slight handwritten markings: "Love is everywhere, and I am loving and lovable." "You are wonderful." "I love you." (unknown authors) These are all billed as positive self-affirmations we should often use for ourselves, according to Hay.

Louise L. Hay's book teaches about the power of the thought becoming your future. I believe that positive thoughts became Keith's (and mine also) way of dealing with his cancer journey— using his brain to think himself healed and envision a future with no cancer. Plus, living life to the fullest.

In Hay's book, she also talks about how "forgiving and releasing resentment", (2005, 7), can help resolve health problems such as cancer. Based on my many years with Keith and our great conversations about his relationships with his parents and ex-relationships, this is my opinion. But I believe he resented losing his father to cancer, but I don't think he resented caring for his mother at the care center (where he often visited her). I feel that his most significant resentment and hurts came from his ex-relationships, where his partners hurt him badly enough that I don't think he could bring himself to forgive them. Perhaps he was working on forgiving those hurts and resentments.

As Louise L. Hay states, "How foolish for us to punish ourselves…because… long ago past." (2005, 7) She goes on to say, "…dissolve... resentment now. Don't wait until you are under the … surgeon's knife." (2005, 7)

"We need to choose to release the past and forgive everyone, ourselves included." "The past cannot be changed. The future is shaped by our current thinking," as Hay says. (2005, 7)

Again, the author's words explain it all. "Love is the miracle cure. Loving ourselves works miracles in our lives." (Hay, 2005, 17)

I believe Keith used this line from the book to guide his cancer journey. "Whatever I choose to believe becomes true for me." (Author unknown) This affirmation is a well-known saying.

As I reviewed the book further, I saw another passage still in the forgiveness section that Keith had marked with his little cute handwritten brackets at both ends that no doubt reminded him to reread this passage once again. "Sometimes, the little kid in us needs to have revenge before it is free to forgive." (Hay, 2005, 71) I bet Keith raised his arms up toward the sky and yelled, "Yes, revenge!" Perhaps Keith was dealing with revenge for the bad exes and his parental loss.

The passage went on to explain a "revenge" (Hay, 2005, 71) exercise. The exercise gave an example of closing one's eyes and thinking of people that person wants to forgive. Then, figure out how those people will win forgiveness and imagine it happening. Perhaps Keith did this? At least, I believe, he read about it.

Then the exercise moved to the "forgiveness" exercises (Hay, 2005, 70). I imagined Keith closing his eyes and concentrating on forgiveness for all who had wronged him. The training goes on to guide in a "visualization" exercise also. I prayed that Keith was finally able to be free from the binds of these hurts.

After all those exercises, one is supposed to be a lot more full of love and able to heal themselves.

"There is so much love in your heart that you could heal the entire planet....for now, let us use this love to heal you." (Hay, 2005, 73)

The best description I can give about Keith's thinking is that he was a Superman at positive thinking. He would still be in a positive mood even while carrying a bag of poison pumping into his veins every few minutes. He had to endure that bag of chemotherapy for forty-two hours after sitting at the oncologist's office for hours receiving his first chemotherapy infusion. When asked how he was doing, he would simply reply, "I'm fine, and I will feel better once this bag comes off, and I will even be better!" Wow!

Louise Hay's book discusses how when someone thinks hard about something like they are worried about receiving bills that they will have to pay and dwell on it, they will receive even more invoices. What we think about, we attract.

The same can go for healing the body. People can worry so much and become afflicted if they constantly think of contracting a disease or disorder. In contrast, if one is not focusing on their sickness but instead believing and feeling like a healthy state, free of physical problems, and concentrating on healing thoughts, they create that healthy mind and body. Keith and I both worked with this attitude often. We placed thoughts out there about cancer cleared out and gone from Keith's body. Then, as a result, during the eleven-year cancer journey, Keith would only experience usually one or two cancer lesions at a time. And, usually, these lesions would be decreased with chemotherapy to a size that could be treated with RFA or ablated. The doctors, early on, would tell Keith that colon cancer usually produces a multitude of cancerous lesions. And many times, too many to control if chemotherapy does not rid them.

I believe Keith, by his thoughts, kept the count and, most of the time, the size of the cancer lesions/tumors to a minimum. Keith's thoughts kept him living for over eleven years.

Still going through the *You Can Heal Your Life* book, (Hay, 2005) I find another section tagged about creating new changes in new thoughts and words. Persons should use the highly recommended positive thoughts rather than negative thoughts. I know Keith used this method because we talked about it often with each other and other people. Keith also learned this with his sound and color healing therapy sessions (more on these subjects later on). With eyes closed, he reported that he would envision a white light going through his body and clearing out the cancer. In his "mind's eye" vision, he would also see each cancer cell dying and washing out through his feet and going to the earth, not to harm again.

Another excellent tidbit of Louise Hay's reads, "… The body is always talking to us if we will only take the time to listen. Every cell within your body responds to every single thought you think and every word you speak." (Hay, 2005, 123)

A month after the cancer-free celebration, Keith was in for a follow-up CT. Next is Keith's report:

In May 2010, during one of my follow-up appointments, doctors found that I had developed a hernia at the colostomy site. I needed another operation to install mesh into my muscle wall to keep my colon inside my body.

On May 18, 2010, I had my hernia repaired, and I am doing very well at this time. It has been ten weeks since the surgery, and I am just starting to get back to being myself with all the activities I used to do.

Before Keith's surgery for the hernia repair, we wanted to grab another dose of JOY. We managed to attend the Avalon Ball on the Saturday just before the abovementioned surgery (which was on the following Tuesday).

Keith was just getting back some energy and stamina, so we danced as much as he could and sat and watched the rest of the time. Just being there seemed to help bring joy to both of us. The search for Joy drove us throughout the years—being able to dance in between the chemotherapies and surgeries and procedures. **We**

strived to keep Joy in our lives as much as possible.

We were new at this cancer-fighting business, flying by the seat of our pants and going by whatever the doctors told us. I was always in the research mode through the years, but I began more extensive research when this cancer happened.

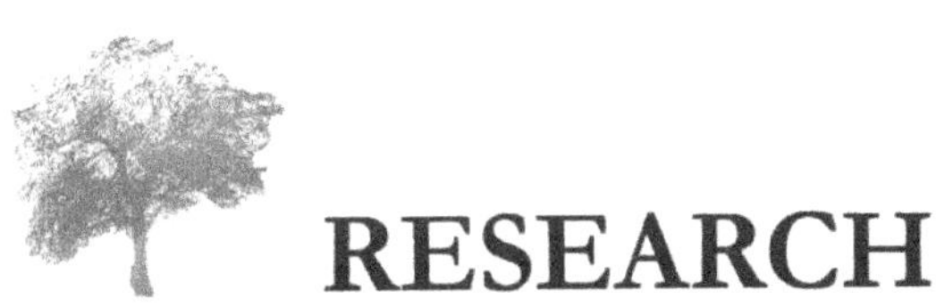# RESEARCH

"Knowledge is power!" —Thomas Jefferson

After the initial shock of Keith's cancer announcement, fear sent me into research mode as I was bound and determined to help Keith fight the demon invading his body.

To tell the truth, we were both surprised about Keith's diagnosis of colon cancer. Given that I considered Keith the healthiest of our pairing, it was surprising he was afflicted. We thought he was very healthy because he ate giant fresh cabbage and vegetable salads five out of seven days a week, plus utilizing the stairs constantly in the high-rise buildings where he worked.

My research revealed more. Keith did not have all the usual risk factors: eats red meats and processed meats a lot (we rarely ate red or processed meats), physical inactivity (Keith was active all day, every day, plus we danced many times a week on top of everything), smoking (Keith never smoked), alcohol (occasional only), diabetes (none), polyps(?).

But, alas, the lack of a colonoscopy was attributed to not detecting cancer in the early stages and perhaps more treatable period of time. Keith revealed later that he had a feeling something was just not right inside his body, but he kept denying there was a problem. He told me he learned a lesson to pay attention to his body, and he recommends that approach to everyone.

Research was our constant companion. Keith rarely did any research. Let me clarify that last statement. Keith researched a lot but on subjects far removed from cancer so that he could "get away" from "that" subject and keep positive. He was the person trying to hold it together by all means possible. I was the project researcher liberally applying dry-eye drops so that I could spend umpteen hours scouring website after website for information on colon cancer metastasizing to the liver. After an important meeting with doctors and with the latest report in hand, I would come home and sit down and research every medical word or term until the message in the information could be understood in laymen's terms.

As you will read in Keith's Story, once I researched, I shared it. I shared the information I found with family and our ever-faithful, good-thought provokers and superior prayer friends. They wanted to be kept in the loop about the cancer journey.

During one of my long research sessions, I found some interesting facts about cancer research. According to the American Cancer Society and Siddhartha Mukherjee, M.D., in his book entitled *The Emperor of All Maladies* (2011, 47), it all began with Hippocrates (460-370 B.C.), the well-known Greek physician. He came up with the language of "carcinos" or "karcinos" and "carcinoma" regarding tumors that were ulcerous or non-ulcerous. Hippocrates was considered the "Father of Medicine." Check out the link for more information about cancer history in the glossary under Cancer History.

Continuing my lengthy research session, Per Siddhartha Mukherjee, M.D.'s book, *The Emperor of all Maladies* (2011, 15-

16), Rudolph Virchow was the founder (1845) of cellular pathology and the first word for cancer, "leukaemia." Virchow's pathology theories evolved from the belief that if a cell grows from another cell, then development can happen "only two ways: either by increasing cell numbers or by increasing cell size." He theorized that cancer is "pathological hyperplasia." Which is the "uncontrolled growth of cells," and "Uncontrollable pathological cell division."

By 1937 the only way to handle cancer was to remove it with surgery or destruct the cancer with radiation. In July 1937, the "National Cancer Institute Act" was passed by congress and signed by President Roosevelt. This act created the new cancer research group, the NCI (National Cancer Institute). But with a second world war at hand, funding and work on the cancer front were virtually stalled for the next ten years. Then, in 1947, Sidney Farber, an American pediatric pathologist, set about working on leukemia, a blood cancer primarily affecting the very young. At that time, chemotherapy did not exist. Farber's friend, chemist Yellapragada Subbarao, joined Lederle Labs and set about uncovering the chemical structure of folic acid. "Yella," as they called him, found that blocking or locking could be achieved by binding to the receptors on the cell. Then the manmade folic acid could be used as an "Antagonist." Yella then shipped Farber his new "anti-folate" to give to leukemia patients. Farber tried the first batch, but it did not work. Yella kept up the research and later sent another batch, which Farber administered to the children suffering from leukemia. This time it worked tremendously well and sent most patients into remission. A manmade chemical halted cancer! Although it would not be known as chemo-therapy for some time, the anti-folate chemical discovery should be considered the first chemotherapy. (Emperor of All Maladies, 2011, 25,27,31,33)

But wait, Paul Ehrlich of Leipzig, Germany, and Robert Koch discovered the cause of tuberculosis. Ehrlich went on to test chemical compounds, and using "chemotherapy" to heal the cancered body parts was "conceptually" born. Siddhartha Mukherjee, M.D. (2011,

84-85)

Fifty years after significant cancer research began in the United States, we found that now, in the 2020s, the cancer survival rate has increased thirty-six percent for those surviving five years or more. More people are receiving their screenings and catching cancer early. Plus, the anti-cancer therapies availability is rising. (article "The War on Cancer turns 50" by Sari Harrar, published AARP Bulletin Nov 2021)

Back to Keith's Cancer Journey

ALONG WITH RESEARCH, hindsight would have been good to have back at the beginning of this cancer journey. If we had known what we know now, we would have secured Keith a referral to the City of Hope at the start. Perhaps the liver ablation that Keith notes below could have been done through the skin, percutaneously, and Keith wouldn't have had yet another open-up surgery. Let's see what Keith had to say next:

This story starts where the first one left off. After being free for a few months, I went in for a regular CT scan in August of 2010, and they saw two new spots on my liver! I made an appointment with the liver surgeon, and he saw me right away.

Because the CT scan could not tell us if these spots were active or not, I needed to get a PET scan. Well, after the PET scan, these two spots showed active. The doctor told us that this is a wonderful thing! How can finding cancer for a second time be a wonderful thing?

Well, the doctor says, there could have been ten spots and not just the two! We told him that was true, but there should have been zero! In our view, zero would have been a wonderful thing!

We decided to have these two spots ablated in late September of 2010. The operation was set for September 23 at ten a.m. The doctor told us that he would cut a T at the top of the original operation scar and ablate the spots with minimal entry into my body.

The day of the operation came, and the time was moved up to seven a.m. Better for me and better for the doctor. I got there at six a.m. to check in, and I got my bed, and they set me up for the operation.

There were a few problems since not everyone knew of the operation change. The change meant that the nurse was not available until later, so my prep was a little late in getting started. I know that because they were wheeling me into the operating room before they got the knockout drugs into me.

Interesting that I got to see the staff getting things ready for me before the operation. I heard later that the assisting doctor showed up at nine for the normal operation, and they had to hold me there until he showed up. My wife was undoubtedly worried by this time because of the extended operation time.

As it turned out, I was in the operating room for over three hours, and the actual operation only took one hour. I woke up in the recovery room, and then they moved me to intensive care, where nobody could sleep. If I moved, one or more of the alarms attached to me would go off and wake up my wife and myself. So, we did not sleep that first night. The second night my wife went home to get sleep, and they moved me down to First Surgical, which is the best place to go if you have to stay in the hospital.

The stay in the hospital was like all the other stays, very unwanted. There is no way people can get better in the hospital. People need to be home to get better and to heal faster. I went in on Tuesday and left the hospital on Saturday.

I was a little amazed that when I saw the operation incision, it was entirely across my body! What happened to the little T at the top of the other incision? I now had a road map on my belly and not just a railroad track. Wow, what an incision.

When I went back to see the doctor in a week, the nurse took out the staples. There were thirty-three altogether, so much for the tiny scar. The nurse insisted on removing the staples. She told me that the doctor is ruthless in ripping them out "willy nilly," causing pain (he is used to the patient being under anesthesia).

After a few weeks, I was able to go back to work, and of course, I had to start CHEMO again. We set Chemo up for the first Thursday in December of 2010 (Comptosar). My last two rounds of Chemo were done on a Monday with three days of the week lost and sometimes the entire week. This time we decided to do the Chemo on Thursday and lose only two days from work. This timing worked very well for the next six months that I was on Chemo.

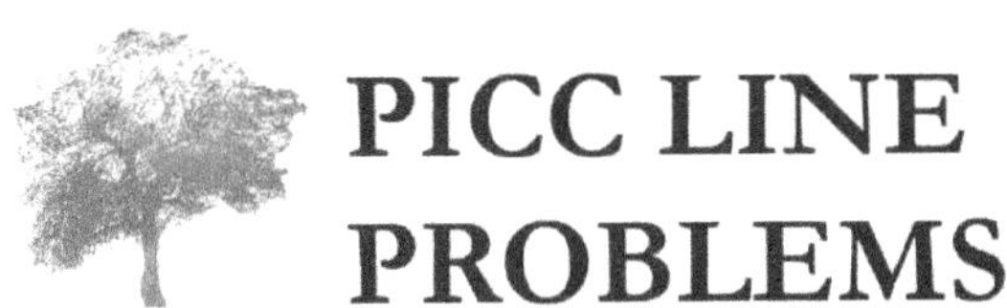# PICC LINE PROBLEMS

B*efore the Comptosar chemotherapy sessions started, doctors placed a PICC line in my right arm the day after Thanksgiving, and my first Chemo was the following week (December). Like before, we had to have it flushed once a week.*

This meant having a nurse come to the house and flush the line for me every other Saturday. This turned out to be a real problem. Not only was my Saturday messed up by this nurse coming by, but she would complain about the Chemo nurse and how she would dress the PICC line on the other weeks. I started calling this the PICC line wars! Each nurse would dress the PICC line differently and then complain about how the other one was doing the job.

The problem became that each one started overdoing it, and the line started to come out of my arm. On the tenth Chemo (two left), the line was out a little more than two inches.

Now, I had to talk the home nurse into flushing the line because she would not do it without the line being reset. With two Chemo sessions left, she wanted me to put a new PICC line? There was no way that was going to happen. The home nurse did the flush, and it was plugged (according to her). She indeed had to push the syringe seemingly hard to get the flush done.

Tuesday night, I had my wife flush it again to see if I, in fact, needed to have this line reset. My wife did the flush with no effort at all. Truth be told, it was so easy that even the Chemo nurse said how much better the line responded than it had in the past.

The last two Chemo sessions went very smoothly, and the line was pulled out after the last one. I would say to you out there that it is much better to have your spouse do the PICC line flush if you can. PICC line wars are the pits.

Keith wrote in his journal about a CT scan report he received while he still received chemotherapy infusions—*Two weeks before the PICC line wars were over, the doctor had me do another CT, and it showed another spot!!!! How could that be??? I am still on chemo!! Why would there be another spot??? I was going crazy, and the doctor told me that this is one of the ablated sites.*

We had the surgeon look at the spot, and he said that I needed to do a PET scan to make sure. Doctors are crazy. Why can't they just tell you the truth and stop doing all these tests? My blood tests made me crazy. My latest blood test showed my tumor marker to be 4.5, and normal for me was 1 to 2.

The doctor told me that it was high because of the Chemo; how can that be? I have been on Chemo for six months and the highest it has ever been was 1.7. Okay, I went and had another blood test after the Chemo, and like the doctor said, my tumor marker was back down to 1.4.

Okay, so what about the new spot? Another CT scan showed the exact location, but it was now seen as stable! All my sites were now stable, meaning that the doctor was right, and this new spot had been ablated. My next appointment is after the 4th of July. The appointment is where they will set me up with another CT scan and

After that CT, a PET scan was scheduled in late July and noted in Keith's Journal: *July 27, 2011, I was in for the PET scan, which showed an increased lesion size found in the March scan. At this point, the liver surgeon did not want to go back into my liver to remove or ablate this new tumor. The doctors decided to have the tumor in the left side of my liver treated with Yttrium Y90 radioactive beads. They would administer the Yttrium through a tube inside one of my arteries in the groin area. In October, another CT was done to view this enlarged tumor that had grown. The CT also showed another lesion on the right side.*

Y90 YTTRIUM MOLECULAR BEADS/ RADIOEMBOLIZATION

As you will read below in Keith's own words, Keith says it took mapping of five hours, which is about right, but then on the date that they inserted the Y90 (Nov 9th), that was a grueling time both for him, the doctors, and me.

In case you are not aware, mapping in the body is when they go in and map out the arteries' roadway to traverse and insert the Y90 Yttrium molecular beads. While mapping, the doctor technicians used certain types of coils to place via an angiogram catheter in the groin area leading to the liver.

They mapped all the liver arteries to and from and embolized or blocked off those arteries going to other organs so that when the doctors administered the Y90, it would not flood and harm those fragile areas. The main focus of this procedure was to give the tumor itself the concentrated radiation beads and overtake and kill all the cancer cells in that tumor.

I wasn't inside the operating room with Keith. I was alone in a tiny waiting area far away, and it seemed like forever. It was the very first time the doctors performed a Y90 procedure at Torrance Memorial Hospital, and the doctors and technicians had to configure things as they went along, so it took time. Keith reported that they had a person from the Yttrium company, with a Geiger counter, inside the specially fitted room running tests the whole time the doctors were doing the procedure. It wasn't two hours, and it wasn't five. It was more like seven or eight hours that I waited and waited. Finally, Keith was through the ordeal and moved to a room. I was lucky to get to see him afterward. The side (of his body) where they placed the radioactive beads was facing the wall, and no one was allowed on that side of the bed. In fact, I couldn't be very close to him while in the room and could not stay but a short time in the room. I made quick visits across the room with small, light, quick hugs and kisses (on the left side).

Keith had to be in the back seat farthest from me to drive him home. And at home, he slept alone and used a separate bathroom for the next two weeks. We couldn't be in close proximity while in the house either.

The joke to everyone (because, again, that is how we handled things, making jokes, having fun, keeping it light) was that Keith was really Superman now that he had the radioactive beads inserted, and he glowed in the dark! I kept checking at night when the lights were all out!

On October 27, 2011, a mapping of the liver was done to ensure none of the Y90 beads made their way into other major areas of the body.

This mapping had me on the CT table for about five hours until all the essential arteries were blocked. That way, the Yttrium would stay on the left side of the liver. On November 9th, the doctors inserted the Y90 into the left lobe of my liver, which took about two hours.

Then about seven hours in recovery before I was able to go home. I had to spend two weeks isolated from other people to make sure people around me would not pick up the radioactive radiation from my liver.

A month later, Keith's doctor scheduled him for a percutaneous RFA (radiofrequency ablation) on one small remaining cancer lesion that the doctors thought had some cells still alive. Here is what Keith said in his journal entry: *On December 8, 2011, I had a small lesion in my liver's right side ablated through the skin with a very long needle with three internal needles. This ablation allowed me to go home the same day after a four-hour recovery. I was able to stay off of any treatment until March of 2012.*

Keith was truly amazing! Just six days later, his company scheduled a retirement party for him in one of their large rooms on the property in Glendale. After the doctors scheduled the March dangerous operation for Keith, Keith decided it was time to retire and put everything into kicking the cancer out of his body.

Keith's energy level and emotions at the retirement party evening were high as he met with everyone as they entered the room. We set up an area for his interviews with guests, and I filmed it all for posterity. A significant number of persons appeared with gifts, hugs, and kind congratulatory words for Keith, and Keith was greatly uplifted and very happy. I was enormously proud that he received so many kudos for his immense thirty-six years of service. An excellent achievement indeed!

New Year's 2012 began with a big sigh of relief. The relief that Keith would no longer have the drive to work (and get up at o-dark thirty) and the exhausting days. We hoped this would give Keith more time to regroup and grow stronger. With the Y90 treatment and ablation behind us, Keith had nothing until a CT and PET scan in March. Meanwhile, we concentrated on keeping him healthy.

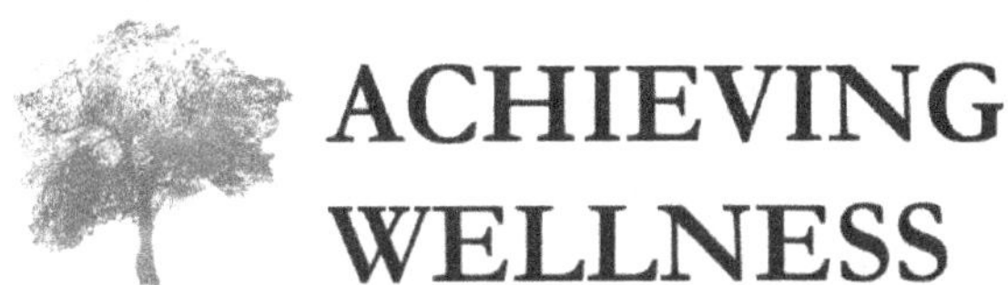

ACHIEVING WELLNESS

Staying healthy while waiting to be cured of cancer was a daunting task for Keith. Balancing healthy living while being bombarded by chemical warfare was a reality that I was always concerned with during the eleven years Keith spent fighting.

Keith was already in excellent shape because he constantly climbed the stairs at the high-rise office buildings where he worked. Plus, with our ballroom dancing many times a week (when Keith didn't receive chemotherapy), Keith had plenty of exercises. These workouts were beneficial to us both, but more so for Keith during his cancer journey. The dancing was a perfect aerobic exercise to help keep Keith fit. Additionally, the endorphins produced by all the activity would help him feel good and send happiness to his brain.

Keith and I had been ballroom dancing since 2002, with our favorite dances being the swing, lindy hop, and balboa. We danced to speedy music played while others sat it out. So, yes, Keith got plenty of physical exercises.

Staying healthy also meant eating healthy. Of course, we

researched the subject and found plenty of people coming to us with their recommendations. But what it came down to was making sure Keith ate well-balanced meals when he felt like eating. Chemotherapy mostly meant limited food since nausea was usually at play with the senses.

Now, with chemotherapy came nausea. In all the years that Keith was receiving the different chemotherapies, he hardly ever had to throw up. He was an early learner on wearing wristbands made for motion or seasickness and increasing the band's tightness according to how he felt. It was interesting to see that these bands worked well to stave off nausea. An area on the insides of the bands pressed against the wrists. The location was at pressure point P-6, also known as Neiguan. Keith would apply more pressure on that particular area by tightening the bands. This action turned off nausea. To learn more on how this works, you can find information on the Sloan Kettering Cancer Center website link located in the Glossary section under Sloan Kettering. We were both happy that these bands worked well for Keith. Cleaning up vomit was not our favorite duty, to be sure.

Another method that Keith devised for himself that helped keep nausea at bay was forcing himself to eat something small every two hours. Frequent eating is much like what doctors recommend for pregnant women who experience nausea. Doctors suggest eating crackers or something else every few hours to help fight the waves of nausea. This method also works for nausea from chemotherapy treatments. As mentioned, we kept small containers of quick and easy foods that Keith could easily handle for his many feedings throughout the day and night.

Something that Keith found out early was not to eat his favorite food while on chemotherapy and nausea gnawing at his gut. I remember reading this advisory early on, and I pointed it out to Keith because his favorite food was In-N-Out Double-Double and fries (which he had not eaten very often).

Well, in his early experience with chemotherapy, we had gotten another favorite food just after one of his treatments. We thought he was fine but soon found out that was not the case, and the favorite did not stay down. After that, he began to figure out about the bands (after I studied the subject online and bought him his first bands to try) and he figured out how to manage his nausea problems. And, lesson learned—no more favorites consumed after infusions. Otherwise, the favorite would no longer be desired at all.

Unless, that is, your infusions don't cause nausea. Later in the years, Keith's chemotherapy treatments were changed (once again), and this time nausea did not bother Keith at all. I remember the first day after the infusion, and reluctantly I asked him what he thought he could tolerate for lunch. He relayed that he was starving and wanted a big, fat hamburger. Well, being the voice of reason, I picked up a healthy lunch for home, and Keith devoured it all. After so many years of dealing with him eating tiny amounts all day, this was a total change.

The body needs proper nutrition to keep it strong because chemotherapy constantly kills good cells along with the cancer cells. Good nutrition keeps building the cells to keep up the fight.

When Keith could tolerate eating more, we reasoned that well-balanced nutrition for him was proteins; fat; dark, colorful vegetables; fruits; and grains, while keeping sugar and spicy foods as much as we could out of the diet. We always aimed for longevity foods such as fungi (mushrooms), sweet potatoes, tubers, and root vegetables and known anti-cancer foods such as onions, garlic, broccoli, spinach, green beans, beets, Brussels sprouts, radishes, and cauliflower. We read labels to be sure we were buying non-GMO products. I don't care how well the big companies purport that genetically modified and Glysophate-sprayed food products are okay. In our opinion, it just cannot be suitable for humanity or animal. One must wonder if these products have played a significant role in the exponential rise in cancer since they began the GMO (genetically modified organisms) process and pesticide spraying, back when they started to grow bigger crops with fewer bugs.

Another food item that we changed in the past eleven years is the use of real butter. Before butter, we always thought we were doing our health good by purchasing alternatives to butter. They tasted fine and all, but once we found out that alternative types of butter are really made of petroleum products, we changed back to the real thing. However, we started buying butter from the UK, Ireland, or Denmark because of their higher-quality products. Because of what American farmers do with the cows (hormones and antibiotics), we prefer to buy Irish or Danish butter.

Although Keith was the family barbequer and loved his rare steak perfectly seared, (in that he rarely had red meat) he became exceptional at handling a wild salmon (with butter, dill, salt, and pepper) barbecued on a soaked cedar plank. The omega-3 in the fish was essential in rebuilding his destroyed cells. Eating more fish of all types was beneficial for Keith's health and well-being. But of course, we had to know to stay away from mercury-laden fish.

Along with healthy nutrition, it was also essential to keep Keith well hydrated. Gatorade was one of his primary fluids he imbibed often. The doctors recommended this drink to replace electrolytes lost. Water, of course, was essential. We bought mountain-fed spring bottled water and had a filter for the house tap water. Keith found that some bottled water's PH levels that he tested (mostly those reverse-osmosis types) were below the acceptable levels of 6.5-8.5. We noticed that they were selling alkaline bottled water. Those are in the 8.0-9.0 range and claim to solve health problems. At one point, we looked into a home filtration system that would allow us to change the PH level of the water for either drinking water or cleaning water. Since it was pretty expensive, we chose to pay medical bills instead.

A serious issue that we had to deal with regarding keeping Keith healthy for the cancer fight was dealing with the physical changes Keith was going through. Doctors had warned us early on that Keith would lose his hair and have to deal with keeping his weight up for his strength. In preparation, Keith bought many newsboy caps. The same type of hats that the newsboys of the early 1900s wore to sell newspapers in the streets. Keith loved these hats and wore them, even though he never wholly lost his hair.

Keith's hair thinned out a lot, and he lost a lot of body hair, including sporadic hair off of his big, bushy eyebrows. He took care of the thinning hair by wearing his newsboy caps. But I never saw a greatly diminished thinned hairline on Keith. I knew Keith felt self-conscious about his eyebrows, so I learned how to "fill in" the brows so they looked more even for special occasions.

One last item to address regarding health is germs. We were not complete germaphobes, but we did our best to keep germs away from invading Keith and causing sickness. Long before the COVID-19 virus, we made sure we had the wiping, sanitizing towelettes with us everywhere, wiping down everything we were going to touch. Plus, we wore face masks before they were in fashion. Keith had a chance of contracting germs readily, so protection was the name of the game continuously. He could not chance getting ill with something else while he had a weakened immune system. Keith did so well that during his entire eleven-year cancer journey, he only came down with a regular cold or allergies a few times. He was very fortunate. As you will see, moving forward, a spiritually healthy body was significant as well.

Keith's spiritual well-being became one of the most essential ventures during the entire cancer journey. Keith utilized many ways to keep his mind, body, and soul intact. Read about these ways next.

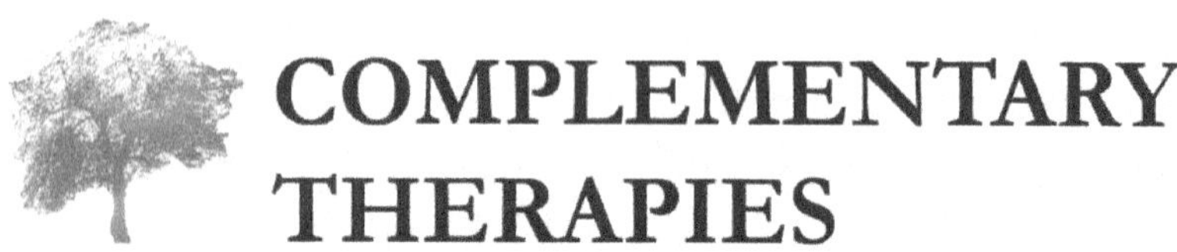# COMPLEMENTARY THERAPIES

In our ever-vigilant quest to ensure that Keith was in the best of health for his fight against cancer, we pulled from those we knew to locate support in a field referred to as alternative or complementary method therapies to Western medicine.

Now, first of all, no, we did not turn solely to alternative medicine instead of what was being offered by the doctors and medical facilities. We just felt that if there were something additional that we could do to help Keith survive the fight of his life and promote wellness, we would pull out all the stops and give it a try. We wanted to be sure he had all the advantages possible.

With Keith's prodigious attitude, he wanted to get back to his good ole life, and he would try almost anything offered. Keith always worked from a positive position, no matter what. This was no different when he was lying in his uncomfortable hospital bed and so miserable after having had his first surgery where they had sliced and diced his colon. I told Keith that a friend of mine offered to help treat him with Qigong. We did not know whether this friend would show up at the hospital, or when, or what he would do. But in our hearts, we felt hopeful and prayerful that it would help Keith. We thought God had sent this angel to Keith's aid, and the time could not come soon enough.

Qigong

ACCORDING TO WIKIPEDIA, "Qigong is a centuries-old system of coordinated body posture and movement, breathing, and meditation used for the purposes of health, spirituality, and martial arts training. With roots in Chinese medicine, philosophy, and martial arts, qigong, traditionally viewed by the Chinese and throughout Asia as a practice to cultivate and balance qi (pronounced "chi," sounding like "chee"), translated as 'life energy.'

"Qigong practice typically involves moving meditation, coordinating slow-flowing movement, deep rhythmic breathing, and a calm meditative state of mind. People practice Qigong throughout China and worldwide for recreation, exercise, relaxation, preventive medicine, self-healing, alternative medicine, meditation, self-cultivation, and training for martial arts." (Wikipedia)

In their exploration of the use of Qigong in cancer care, the NCBI (National Center for Biotechnology Information) stated, "The broad concept of Qigong may be sub-classified as spiritual, healing, medical, or martial Qigong." With the healing Qigong received as external or internal Qigong. Internal via meditative and energy-deriving ways and external Qigong involving moving energy via a skilled practitioner.

Further, the Qigong exercise, Tai Chi, involves postures, breathing techniques, focused thoughts in meditative flowing movements for the move, and flow of vital energy.

NCBI goes on to say, "Energy theory purports that we possess a vital life energy known as Qi (pronounced chee). We are born with a quantity of essential Qi to begin life....To sustain life, we replenish our vital energy by accumulation of nutritive Qi through meditation, exercise, the foods and herbs we ingest, the water we drink, the air we breathe, and, even possibly, more importantly, our emotional and belief states. The postulate that <u>mindset can influence health</u>, healing, and longevity is a root tenet of Chinese medicine….Disease is attributed to stagnation or blockages of this vital energy flow."

And then, very soon, Dean-O appeared at my husband's bedside, offering calm in an otherwise unnerving hospital environment. I disappeared in the hallway to not disrupt anything, plus I wanted to be there to ward off any hospital staff from interrupting the session.

Observing the room from the hallway, I could see that Dean-O held a nice-size, clear, crystal, quartz, smooth, round stone in the open palm of his hand. I watched from afar as Dean-O held the globe just above the areas of Keith's body. He deliberately and slowly moved the hand-held crystal globe while quietly speaking as needed. During this process, I remembered that quartz crystals have healing attributes. So, I was not altogether surprised that Dean-O used this stone for the treatment. On Dean-O's way out, after asking him if I could compensate him for the treatment, Dean-O responded that he had already received his payment from serving Keith.

And so, it started back in 2009—the complimentary complementary cancer Qigong treatments. They were complementary to the medical treatments and complimentary because of Dean-O's great heart. As I learned early on, Dean-O is a gentle soul with pure and genuine benevolence constantly pouring from him.

Fast-forward years later, a letter from Dean-O came today, September 14, 2020. I was lucky to locate him once again. I was assembling *Keith's Story* and wanted to include his segment.

I first got to know Dean-O years ago, back at my last job. Dean-O would cheerfully appear often at my office door for a chat. Just after Keith had his first surgery and was still in the hospital, Dean-O happened by the office, and I informed him about Keith's surgery. He must have sensed the worry flowing from me. Because, without hesitation, he asked if it would be okay to see Keith.

I knew Dean-O practiced Qigong, which might help Keith recover and fight against the cancer attacking his body. I was glad Dean-O could see him at the hospital right away. That set the stage, and Dean-O started coming to the house once Keith was home and continued to guide and treat him for a number of years.

These treatments and guidance sessions were instrumental in assisting Keith with his healings from surgeries and chemotherapies. After all, they had given Keith a few months to live, and here, years later, with Dean's guidance and treatments, Keith was doing well in his cancer journey.

After reading about our faith and religious beliefs, a person might be wondering how we came to believe that Qigong would be beneficial for Keith. I sensed that some people might not be fully aware or have knowledge about Qigong (as well as Tai Chi). Keith and I were very open and receptive to the Qigong sessions since we saw absolutely no contradictions with our religious endeavors. In fact, we saw Qigong as an enhancer, a healing, and easily coexisted with our faith beliefs.

Here is Dean-O's letter of September 14, 2020:

Aloha!

I believe what I did for Keith first was to do very basic forms to see how he would respond to what I was trying to do for him. The beginning forms I did with him were to teach him the portals of energy in his hands, feet, and the top of his head. We had to get him used to receiving and dispersing energy through those portals. Once accomplished, I was able to teach him how to store energy in his lower Dantian. This lower Dantian area is about two to three fingers below the navel. As we progressed, I felt that he was very sensitive to the energy. That was such a positive sign for me as it was for Keith.

As time went on, I used many different forms to help Keith use his mind, body, and spirit to help him recover. Love & Aloha! Dean-O

Later, Dean-O also wrote: *Qigong is a practice for balance in our lives. We've been taught to use Qigong to help ourselves first. Then we were taught the different healing styles to help ourselves and others.*

Qigong moves energy through the body, keeping good positive energy within and exhausting the bad energy out to, let's say, the earth as one example. It can move energy through organs (solid and hollow) to clear and rid them of bad energy.

At this point, I might interject thoughts about mindset and Keith. During Keith's entire cancer journey, Keith's mindset was the key factor for his survival. Even if he were not having a good day, he would muster a positive mindset. I know he derived his mindset from his positive thinking as well as his therapies and activities involving Qigong, Tama-do, Tai Chi, and social dancing.

At one point, Dean-O became overly busy and determined he would need to hand off treatments to Pat, a Tama-do practitioner. She performed her services in a relaxed office environment. Keith would drive to the hour-plus appointments, or I would take him if he weren't up to driving.

Pat knew Dean-O through their studies of Qigong. Pat took over caring for Keith with her Tama-do methods. Each time Keith was treated, it was evident that he experienced more energy and gratitude and fight to take on the subsequent medicinal therapy (chemotherapies, ablations, etc.).

Tama-do

FAST-FORWARD TO SEPTEMBER 2020, when I received an email from Pat after I contacted her and asked if she would write something for *Keith's Story*. Here is her reply:

My Tama-do experience with Keith was and still is a wonderful relationship that I cherish. We learned and taught each other so much as we worked with his health issues. Keith is still helping my clients as I use him (anonymously) as an example of strength, joy, and love for Life.

As a Tama-do Energy practitioner of Sound, Color, and Movement (Qi Gong), Keith was referred to me in 2009. As Keith began his "campaign" to beat cancer with Western/Allopathic medicine, he asked me to be part of his team of health practitioners. Being a complementary practitioner, I helped to round out his team.

Keith came to me because Tama-do Academy is based on science, energy, and spirituality...we work to integrate body, mind, and spirit. Fabien Maman, the founder of Tama-do Academy, is defined in Webster's dictionary as the Father of vibrational sound therapy. Fabien's strict and scientific protocol with sound and cells/human body has led the way in sound therapy and color since the 1980s.

Keith and I worked hard to help keep him strong, balanced, and "dancing" as he went through his treatments of chemotherapy and surgeries. And his dry sense of humor always kept us both laughing and "deadpanning" our way through the challenges of beating cancer. His "Buster Keaton" expression spoke volumes as he came for his weekly sessions. He always left with a smile on his face and an aura and physical body fuller and Lighter. It kept him balanced, relaxed, and hopeful until his next chemotherapy sessions.

I moved my practice to Long Beach in 2016, and the distance kept him from seeing me. But I kept sending love, Light and Chi to both Keith and Mary.

As they say, "Energy can neither be created nor destroyed... it just BE!"

Pat Aoki

310-629-8741

Tama-do-LongBeach.com

www.Tama-do-LongBeach.com

thebluetreecenter@gmail.com

At the start of Pat's treatments, we were very intrigued once we found out how Pat treated Keith with something called Tama-do. Coming from experiencing Qigong, this was a whole new understanding for us. Pat was very kind in explaining the practice, and Keith seemed most receptive to her treatments.

When I searched online for Tama-do, I found the website, simply https://tama-do.com.

Looking further for more assistance in understanding Tama-do, I found this great saying on the website's home page: "The way of the soul to the light." This is Tama-do! According to their website:

In the early '80s, Fabien Maman conducted a revolutionary sound/cellular biology experiment showing for the first time under the microscope, the impacts of acoustic sound on human cells and their energy fields. His findings, documented in spectacularly beautiful slides, changed the landscape of Sound Healing as we know it today.

Further from the Tama-do website, Fabien was many things, including a musician and an acupuncturist. However, instead of needles applied to the command points, Fabien used tuning forks of different calipers, producing sound waves that healed the body with non-invasive techniques.

Fabien studied the astonishing healing effects of sound on the human cells and discovered the sounds' and later color's ability to heal. When we first learned of this amazing therapy, we were astounded. We were always prayerful that this would help save Keith.

After one of Keith's first sessions with Pat, I asked Keith how it transpired and what he experienced. He revealed that Pat would lead him through mental exercises whereby he would envision a vivid, ample white healing light coming into his body, through the top of his head and slowly emanating throughout his body, as it moved down to his feet and out of the bottom of the feet into the ground.

I recalled a day I watched in person while once again I stood outside another hospital room doorway. Pat laid down something on Keith's rumpled hospital bed coverings, then rolled out a fabric container holding a row of musical tuning forks of various sizes. One by one, she took them out and tapped them on the bed frame to make a sound emanate, then applied them to the different meridian points on Keith's body. Keith had once again gone through a challenging surgery and was probably in pain and very miserable but lying there quietly taking in the therapy.

I cannot remember whether Pat used the color scarves that day, but I remember a few group sessions that I joined with Keith, where Pat used color scarves and various sounds. To me, it was akin to meditation (calming) but also invigorating at the same time. I was both relaxed and energized coming from those group sessions.

There would be a time when we happened along an outdoor fair and people selling sound bowls from Asia. Knowing sound had been helping Keith, we would eagerly search for "his" bowls so that he could take them home and work on his sound therapy at home. We ended up with three lovely bowls. Each time he picked them up, the bowls seemed to sing wholeheartedly for Keith. I found that if I tapped the edge first, then pressed on the sides while moving the wooden mallet, the sound worked better. Keith's singing bowls were perfect for his therapy.

Tai Chi

AFTER PAT MOVED OUT of her offices and set up another office too far for Keith to travel there, Keith searched for another therapy. Thankfully, we found the new treatment, Restorative Tai Chi, in our church bulletin, and Keith signed up!

In the beginning, I accompanied Keith to make sure of what he was getting himself into and thought perhaps I would also benefit from this newfound therapy. Newfound for us. Neither of us had attended Tai Chi in our lives.

Just being inside the church (where they held some of the classes) gave me energy. The lessons taught were just inside the church's entryway, and inside the church, the overflow would take place. It was like God was there with us, guiding the ebb and flow of the energies along with us. Each person partaking in the lessons would stand on a pre-marked X area on the carpet. The Xs were pieces of masking tape.

I then figured that the Xs were all spaced out neatly to give each person plenty of movement room. I was glad I was there. Then the lesson began with the moving and swaying of the arms about the body. The warmup included moving the Qi.

Subsequently, Keith would continue to be present for the Tai Chi classes, sometimes going five days/nights a week for the next four years. Tai Chi seemed to enrich Keith's life tremendously. Even if he was going through some tough times with his cancer journey, he made his way to Tai Chi (or I took him), and he came home energized for days. Not only was he energized, but his mental health was also immensely assisted. Tai Chi was helping Keith. Further, surrounded by friends and having people to talk with, Keith aided and elevated his mental well-being.

In researching for more information about Tai Chi, I asked my longtime dear friend to share on the subject. She told me that the slow movements reminded her of Japanese dance. Further, she always thought of Tai Chi as part of Qigong and yoga, attributes for the well-balanced body. She also thought of Tai Chi as Chinese martial art, but she was not interested in it as a martial art but chose to partake because of its health benefits; strengthening balance plus yin/yang balance, breathing, focusing, calming.

Per NCCAM (National Center for Complementary Alternative Medicine), they describe Tai Chi as slow, relaxed body movements and the making of forms, many as animal forms such as the crane. One action flows to the following form without stopping. The slow movements made by persons keep their backs erect and their breathing meditative-like.

Interestingly, I found a study online listed with the U.S. National Library of Medicine under clinicaltrials.gov entitled: *Effect of Tai Chi Vs. Structured Exercise on Physical Fitness and Stress in Cancer Survivors. Check out the online link in the Glossary under Tai Chi Vs. Structured Exercise*

They undertook a study of cancer survivors on how the art of Tai Chi vs. typical aerobic exercise fared in helping them continue to fight against more cancer growth. Since Tai Chi had been used in Asia for thousands of years to support wellness and stress and used to "promote healing by improving the flow of Qi (energy)," it is thought that it should help the Western world with the same.

In visiting the famed MD Anderson Cancer Center online regarding their tagged information about Tai Chi, I found that Tai Chi is an *"effective form of meditation for cancer patients."* Find more information in the Glossary under MDAnderson.

Anderson calls Tai Chi a "moving meditation" with "graceful motions" with the correct breathing and posture that helps promote the body and mind, enhances the immune system, and relieves pain. "Internal balance for a healthy body." (mdanderson.org)

Please take note that through the years, Keith practiced meditation regularly, at home, using his computer and Deepak Chopra's recorded Guide to *Well-Being Meditations*. Keith would find quiet time in the office, place the earplugs, and spend a relaxing time with Chopra's comforting, meditative guiding voice. Since meditation is an excellent way of re-centering oneself, occasionally, I would play the meditations for myself.

In Your Mind

ANOTHER BOOK THAT MY HUSBAND, Keith, studied was *Ageless Body*, Timeless Mind by Deepak Chopra. This book speaks about how the body's cells pay attention to attitudes and what is happening. Should we be going through significant problems like depression or misery, these problems can very well bring on harsh consequences such as cancer or heart problems, thus decreasing life expectancy. It is interesting to note that Keith had gone through tremendous heartbreak and depression, over and over, for many years.

Deepak Chopra writes, "Because the mind influences every cell in the body, human aging is fluid and changeable…." And, "For nothing holds more power over the body than beliefs of the mind." These notions are fantastic, as per the following statement from Chopra's book: "If you change your perception, you change the experience of your body and your world."

When they say, "It's all in your mind," that is part of the equation. Another saying is, "Mind over matter." Change how you view your body, your situation with cancer (or any health problem), and the possibilities are there to change your health.

One way that Deepak Chopra teaches how to improve and change the mind is to master the body through meditation. He instructs that one should be in times of complete silence, be quiet in the mind of thoughts, and connected to the source. Slow breathing is part of the meditative process. But natural management of the breathing becomes automatic. A person breathes in and out through their nose. Breathing deeply, slowly, and regularly calms the body and emotions. Deepak recommends sitting comfortably either on the floor or in a chair. Sit erect with hands relaxed on legs. During meditation, Deepak suggests meditative mantras. Mantras are words or sound repeated many times to change the mindset.

It has always been Keith's belief and my belief that these complementary modalities no doubt played a massive role in Keith's life in retaining him to remain whole longer. Meditation, Qigong, Tama-do, and Tai Chi were all instrumental in serving Keith well; in relieving psychological stress, enhancing his sense of well-being, improving his musculoskeletal functioning, assisting digestion and lung functions, calming, easing his pain, improving his sleep, balancing his energies, and most important of all, balancing and promoting his self-esteem.

I had a feeling that a staunch religious person may read through all the aforementioned complementary ways Keith used to help him through the past eleven years and might question how our religious beliefs fared while using these healing modalities.

Both Keith and I believed in God, and, our major religion we followed was Catholicism. We also prayed about the way we should go and believed that God brought us what was needed for Keith's journey.

We also held a broad, open view of life. We were open to new approaches, new ideas of balancing our lives. We also believed in Buddha's philosophies of life as well as Laozi's Tao-te Ching—"Way of life to restore harmony and tranquility." Read more at the link listed in the Glossary under Tao-de Ching.

Now that I have let you know our methods of helping Keith's spiritual and healthy well-being, we best bestow a bit of advocacy information for your perusal, since a person going through cancer care and those assisting should learn to be advocates early on.

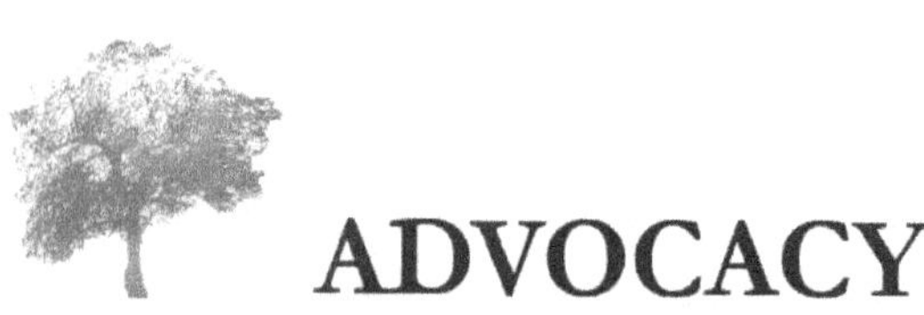

ADVOCACY

Early in the cancer journey process, we learned that we had to study to be our own advocates. When I was not in the room with Keith, he learned self-advocacy. And, when he was unable to make his own decisions, I stepped up to be Keith's supporter, backer, promoter, and protector advocate.

The hardest part of advocacy was to figure out when to stop listening and when to act to make a proper decision. It was difficult ascertaining what to question or what we should ask. I wish we had known. Hindsight. Yes, "wish we had known" became a regular part of a sentence we would say more than a few times. I wish someone had been our advocate as it all started and guided us as doctors told Keith he had dreadful stage 4 colon cancer and given only months to live. I wish someone had advised us we should have sought advice from a key cancer facility before making significant decisions.

But, alas, we had little help initially and, therefore, were forced to become our own advocates for Keith's welfare. We banded together as a powerful unit, willing to do anything needed, go anywhere required, and do pretty much anything to eliminate the cancer from Keith's body.

Over time, both Keith and I learned a lot about advocating for the rights and needs of a cancer patient. Keith had been his mother's advocate for many years, and I had been my parents' and my previous husband's advocate many times, many years, but never for cancer. We both had to learn many lessons along the way.

Becoming Keith's advocate was the path we were to follow. We jumped in with all four feet, hands, and two heads to give the subject our full attention. We raised our hands and asked questions and waited for answers. With answers, we always seemed to have more questions, and so on it went.

Keith kept an ongoing log on his computer of surgeries, procedures, and tests throughout the eleven years while I took notes at every doctor's and specialist's appointment. Nearly every time, I diligently carried my notepad and pen (or iPad later on) to track what they told us. We asked the doctors to decipher any medical terminology unfamiliar to us. And oftentimes coming home and working late into the night, researching every word noted to get a more complete understanding. We knew that we could make more informed decisions for Keith's care and well-being when we understood more.

We would learn about the diagnosis at each turn of the journey and determine the treatments offered. Then we would communicate with the doctors and specialists to understand what to expect before, during, and after each surgery, procedure, test, and treatment. First, we asked what kind of cancer did Keith have and what stage was the cancer? Was there a biopsy/pathology processed, and what did they find? Had the cancer metastasized? Had the cancer spread to other organs? One of the biggest questions we kept asking was, "Can the cancer be killed or cured?" And with the answers to these questions would come more questions, such as, "What are the treatment options?" and "What are the side effects?"

As you will see in *Keith's Story*, you will find plenty of instances characterizing the advocacy used to help Keith survive and thrive during his cancer journey. Oftentimes, our advocacy would save Keith's life.

Thankfully, since dealing with my previous husband's wearying, long-term illness, and subsequent death, I had some medical terminology stored to support our advocacy for Keith. But even with that, I was constantly searching to decipher new jargon for test results and new procedures and cancer therapies. Research and education were constantly ongoing.

We were fortunate during the treatment years that most doctors and specialists we met were well receiving of our endless questions and requests. Furthermore, Keith was always, thankfully, surrounded by doctors who would respond quickly to our sometimes-worrisome queries while we were away from their offices. After leaving a message on the office phone, Keith's oncologist always returned the call speedily. Over at the City of Hope, we were also fortunate to get in touch rapidly with Keith's doctors and specialists. They each had assistants who made sure we had their contact info (including email) so that informing the doctor (via the assistants) of something urgent (or noteworthy) was quick and easy. Their response back to us was always phenomenal!

We recommend the techniques mentioned above to establish a good rapport with your doctors and specialists and if you are unable to do so, request a replacement as this is your life on the line. Further, make sure your oncologist talks with and involves any enmeshed specialists in your treatment plan. With Keith, he had his oncologist, who was in charge of figuring out which chemotherapy to administer. Keith also had the radiologist surgeon who was in charge of taking out the cancer as it appeared. The two of them gathered thoughts and often spoke, planning which processes would take place next.

Getting second opinions and referrals to cancer specialty hospitals is critical if you can. Something we wish we would have done at the beginning of the cancer journey was get a second opinion before starting with chemotherapy. But back then, we were basically "green" regarding cancer. We were both in shock at the cancer news. So, all we knew initially was just go along with what the hospital did. They immediately sent an oncologist to Keith for a consultation at his bedside. That oncologist turned out to be excellent, so we have no regrets. However, please understand that you can get other recommendations for oncologists and cancer care hospitals. You don't always have to go along with what the hospital gives you. We found with Keith's situation that we felt pressured because everyone said to get going with chemotherapy right away. So, we had no time to shop for another oncologist or even think about going elsewhere. Or so we thought.

Ensure that your doctors, oncologists, and specialists take the time you need in your appointments. Bring with you the questions you want answered. Here are some things you might want to ask them: What type of cancer do I have? Carcinoma, lymphoma, leukemia, sarcoma, melanoma? What stage is my cancer? Chances of eradicating, remission, or getting it under control? What is my tumor marker acronym and number, and what does it mean? Does the medical office supply online access to records and test reports? What are the pros and cons of my recent surgery or treatment plan? If you had surgery, ask for the tissue biopsy report and ask if technicians did a liquid biopsy. Also, ask if technicians processed advanced genomic tests and written reports.

Once you learn the type, staging, and tumor marker information for your cancer, you can understand more. A tumor marker is a biological marker that can show the elevated presence of the cancer. Knowing which type of cancer you have and what stage can help you when the doctor tells you your cancer plan. And when it comes to your tumor marker, knowing whether your tumor marker has increased or decreased might help you understand if the treatment is working (sometimes other factors can also affect your tumor marker). And, whatever you do, if they try to paint a grim picture with only months to live, DON'T GIVE UP. NEVER GIVE UP.

Most medical offices have an online capability for you to access parts of your medical chart. These days most companies have it implemented and easy to use. We could easily access the online services for the office staff at Keith's oncologist. We could also view or request a myriad of items; scheduling, appointments, messages to the doctor (like a test report done at the facility he does not have access to), view a lab test completed at a lab, and download signed forms such as lab requests.

As with Providence, another primary medical provider in our area, they have MyChart. That comes in handy for viewing test reports instead of scheduling an appointment with the doctor to have the test results read weeks later.

While on the subject of test results, I would like to point out that The City of Hope was the best in quickly getting Keith's results. Usually, scheduling would be done for all tests plus the doctor's clinical appointment to give the results on the same day as the tests. Yes, Keith would arrive early morning for labs and sometimes either an MRI, CAT test or both. Then, the test results would have been compiled and available for the doctor's appointment by the afternoon. No more waiting for weeks to find out news about Keith's cancer. We usually knew the results the same day as the tests.

Speaking about appointments, be sure to keep all appointments the best that you can. It is within these appointments that your tests may reveal further surgeries or treatments that will prolong your life. So, even though you may not feel your best some days, please do everything you can to make it to the appointments.

One of the patient's advocates' goals is handling insurance proficiently. Usually, this was my job since I wanted to protect Keith from undue stress. From the start, the process of wrangling our testy employer-run insurance carrier was always precarious! They were clearly in the business of making sure they did not pay anything until we fought for the payments. Sometimes I would have to deal with the doctor's office, then the insurance carrier office, then the employer office to get to the bottom of who had dropped the ball on paying the bills.

As you can imagine, there were so many bills another person might just pay them rather than deal with it all. It was something to watch regarding insurance billings: we were often billed quickly and directly from the medical office before they even billed the insurance. They knew it takes time to get paid by an insurance company, so sometimes it was easier for them to bill a client, so they could get paid quicker (and then later also receive money from the insurance company).

On other occasions, companies sent us bills stating they were involved in the surgery or procedure when they were supposed to bill under another doctor because the other doctor was approved under the insurance. I bet many get paid because people are too sick to deal with it. Advocates are needed for these patients to handle such blatant insurance issues.

Thankfully, a few years after Keith retired and enrolled in Medicare, he signed up for unparalleled insurance coverage to supplement the Medicare coverage. Since then, we thankfully never had to deal with any more insurance billing problems.

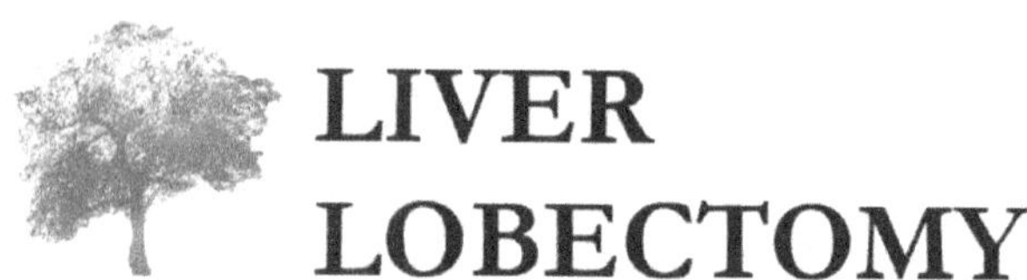# LIVER LOBECTOMY

The CT and PET scan tests on March 1, 2012, revealed that the cancer lesion the Y90 treated back in 2011 had diminished hypermetabolic activity, but live cancer cells were still evident! The Y90 did not entirely work!

In his own words from his journal, Keith will tell you what the doctors decided: *The surgery was set for March 20, 2012. The left lobe to be removed along with nodules (metastases) discovered on the diaphragm. Biopsies were done in both areas; these biopsies showed that it indeed was Colon Cancer and not a new cancer. As a follow-up to the lobectomy, I was placed on Xeloda in pill form.*

This lobectomy on Keith's liver was by far the scariest surgery up to this point. The surgeon removed half of Keith's liver. Surgery on the liver is always extremely dangerous since a person can easily die of severe blood loss quickly. The doctors advised us of the dangers, but we were praying that this surgery would eliminate all of the cancer and end the treacherous ongoing chemotherapy regimen Keith had to endure. We made sure Keith saw our priest, who anointed him with oils and prayers in preparation for his surgery. We always prayed for all involved: the doctors for guiding them to do the proper techniques, for Keith in recovering from the surgery, and yes, Keith said he prayed for me for strength to help him during the process.

The surgery day came, and I will never forget us standing by the door at the hospital and hugging each other tightly. So many surgeries already that left Keith's body scarred and in pain for a lengthy time and we had only gentle side hugs in the past. A bit of kissing and saying our "I Love Yous," and they whisked him off to the OR. The surgery took about five and a half hours. I had gotten used to the doctors telling me one thing, and the time being longer. It always seemed to take much longer for surgeries and procedures than anyone said. Nevertheless, I worried greatly!

After the surgery, Keith was in recovery for a while, then moved to First Surgical. We had made prior reservations with the doctor at the hospital and begged all involved to pull strings to get Keith sent to the First Surgical Ward. That's because it was comparable to a first-class hotel room, except with medical equipment added. It was like being in a museum (with artifacts in the hallways) of huge suites with luxury fold-out beds for wives like me. Good thing, as Keith needed me. This surgery went well, but I cried when I first saw him. The hospital staff installed a C (central) line in his neck.

The C-line is a venous line placed into the large vein. Multiple IV lines came from this C-line, allowing the nurses to administer multiple fluids and meds and make blood draws. This type of setup, we learned, is used in case of a critical need; nurses administer meds or fluids faster than just through a single IV. My first sight of him significantly freaked me out. I saw him laid out flat on his back with his arms to his sides and all kinds of tubes and things coming from him from every which way. His nose had the thing he hated the most—the nasogastric tube going down to his stomach. Oxygen tubes in his nose also. Blood pressure cuff on one arm, the oxygen finger thingy on the other hand. So much going on that he couldn't even scratch his face when he was awake or find the nurse's call button and press it for help. Good thing I was there. Thanks be to God, Keith made it through that challenging surgery.

"Look in the mirror at least once every day, and give thanks for the heart that continues to beat and the invisible force on which those heartbeats depend." (Dr. Wayne Dyer, *Power of Intentions*, p 229)

I remember sleeping there three nights and continually being his advocate, getting him the help he needed day and night willingly. Remembering also having to shush a noisy nurse barreling through the door in the middle of the night, and on another occasion helping Keith complain about a smelly nurse who gave him nausea when she entered the room (she wore too much cologne).

I would be kicked out daily by the early morning crew, who would announce that I had to leave for a bit. Not sure what that was about, but I knew they were changing the team. But they changed the team at night, and I did not leave the room. Every morning, off I would go home, take a quick shower, gather the mail, check messages, get breakfast, and get back to the hospital and go straight to his room.

That would be the routine until he was more stable, and he could use the call button for help on his own. Keith had a heart monitor hooked up to him, and who knows what else. So much that often, if he moved any part of him, the alarms sounded. Sleeping was not an option there. Maybe a bit for Keith because he had pain meds. The fold-out bed was excellent, and they even gave me sheets, blankets, and pillows. I felt like I was in a luxury hotel suite within a hospital. On occasion, they even offered me meals.

Slowly Keith improved, and I was able to sleep at home. I still spent my days with Keith. Keith enjoyed watching the church services on TV. They had a chapel outside the hospital (attached to the hospital) and allowed patients to view the services. Occasionally I would go to the services, where I offered up many more healing prayers for Keith.

Keith's abdomen certainly looked like he had been in one big war. Lots of "train" tracks (he called them) back and forth and up and down. My heart yearned to have him heal quickly and out of pain. There would be no big, tight hugs for a long time.

The operation was on March 20, 2012. A PET scan (a scan to show the hypermetabolic activity of cells—indicating cancer, usually) completed on June 22, 2012, showed NO hypermetabolic activity! God is Great! What a great birthday gift to Keith. Once again, we were on top of the world.

But, darn! We had to pull back the reins a bit when the following PET scan in November gave us disappointing news. Keith wrote about it in his journal here: *November 16, 2012 PET scan reveals a new tumor growing in the liver's remaining right lobe. This tumor was of good size, about 6cm, and was in an area that RFA through the skin could not be done at that time.*

We wanted to get another opinion of this tumor; I was sent to the City of Hope to see what they thought of this new tumor. Another CT was ordered on November 29th with iodine contrast to reveal the blood vessels and their location with the tumor. One of the major vessels was going through the tumor, and another Y90 was suggested.

We were both very disappointed to find new cancer growing in the remaining liver section! Keith had been taking chemotherapy pills Xeloda since his March surgery. Every month he had tumor marker blood tests. Very gradually the counts rose with the last one being at 6.1. For Keith's oncologist, it was not all that alarming. But clearly an indication of the revelation on the recent PET scan.

November 29, 2012, A CAT scan with iodine contrast was completed on Keith to show the major blood vessel within the liver. Weeks dragged on, and finally, the doctors (liver surgeon and oncologist) came to the conclusion that the doctors could not ablate the tumor. The doctors recommend Keith to the City of Hope for evaluation. We were in the middle of December.

I want to mention more about the City of Hope's wonderful campus. Keith had been through the ringer by the end of 2012. He had had appointments and promises by UCLA, with none coming to his assistance. He had meetings with doctors in the Providence region in our area with radiologists promising this and that, but with lots of radiation planned. Then, when the doctors finally recommended Keith to City of Hope just before January 2013, we did have a brand-new sense of real Hope.

Our experience from the start was remarkable. With other doctors, there was always a long wait time for just an office appointment to meet a doctor with many promises to come that never materialized without constant pressure on their offices. However, with City of Hope, we got an appointment within days of our first call. Their campus is enormous. We were guided to the massive main parking lot at the entrance and advised to enter the building by the water fountain.

When we entered, it was confusing, but we were met very quickly by a kind person who probably saw that we looked lost. He guided us to our first check-in area for new patients and promptly took care of Keith. Then another super-friendly, blue-cloaked person (who we figured out later was another volunteer) guided us through the halls up the elevators to another section where Keith had his first appointment with the doctor.

Usually, appointments with specialists are hurried, but not at the City of Hope. Everyone treated us with kindness and care during every meeting. The doctor was superbly the very best. He sat with us and explained, showing us images on a computer, answered questions, even listened to our personal talk, and never hurried us along.

Our opinion is that the doctors involved at the City of Hope and the whole of the City of Hope continuously gave us enormous hope that endured for the next seven years. Keith would not have had seven more years if it wasn't for the City of Hope. We are forever grateful for the kindness, the research, and the skill they show, even down to the cafeteria workers.

The City of Hope was terrific and recommended a Y90 radioembolization on the new tumor. First, doctors scheduled a remapping on January 9, 2013. Keith tells you a bit about that experience: *On January 9th, another mapping was done at the City of Hope, which kept me on the table less than two hours, a three-hour recovery, and I was on my way home. The Y90 was then set to be done on January 24th, which had me on the table for less than an hour; after another four hours of recovery, I was sent home.*

As Keith explained before, on January 24th came the actual insertion and applying the Y90 Yttrium radioactive beads into the tumor. The day began early, driving through the pouring rain from the beach cities to Duarte. Friendly people at the City of Hope greeted us, and technicians tested Keith's blood, and an IV was placed in his arm for what the nurses referred to as a fantastic cocktail they promised later.

Then came his Ticket to Ride (no kidding, it says that on the paperwork) to the radiology surgery room. They readied the surgery room with unique floor mats to catch and contain any tiny radioactive beads that got away.

Again, those on duty spoke about the cocktail and advised Keith to ask for more if he experienced any pain. I was allowed in the pre-op room to witness these interactions. They informed him that he would not be totally out since doctors and technicians would give directions on breathing and moving.

The radiologist surgeon appeared to explain once again how he had isolated the tumor (during the re-mapping phase) with the arteries leading to and from the cancer. The process spared the remainder of the liver. The isolation would lessen the likelihood of liver failure! To worry about this was extremely frightening since Keith only had the remaining half of a liver left!

The doctors and technicians completed the procedure quicker than expected. The staff kept saying that it was the smoothest Y90 procedure they had experienced. It ran so smoothly that they finished earlier than expected—only one and a half hours! Remember when it took seven or eight hours at that other hospital? When the doctor came out to talk to me, I thought something had happened to Keith since it was so soon after they had started.

Three hours later, Keith was released to go home. They sent him home with four prescriptions that included pain meds Keith never took (he had a high pain tolerance and hated to take pain meds) plus two antibiotics to keep him from experiencing any infections. I was able to pick up the prescriptions at City of Hope, so I didn't have to stop at the pharmacy at home. We had a volunteer push Keith's wheelchair a very long way through a vast parking lot to the car because the drive-up area at the entrance was too hectic. We LOVED the City of Hope!

Once I got Keith home, he would be in his separate bedroom and bathroom, and if we sat in the living room, I had to be on the other side, far away from him. We knew the drill—Superman would be glowing again!

Meantime, Keith had a CAT scan scheduled a month and a half later at the City of Hope. The radiologist surgeon warned us that, most likely, at that point, the tumor might show that it had grown because of the Y90 treatment. We had experienced this fright the first time with the previousY90 experience, so we were already forewarned. We honestly enjoyed how this doctor and his assistants told us everything and more to keep us well informed. The doctors advised us they would know whether the Yttrium treatment worked in four to five months.

A month later, Keith started on Vectibix chemotherapy. He had these sessions every other week for twelve/thirteen weeks with short intervals in between for short breaks. Many friends and family asked us, "How long will Keith need to be on chemotherapy?" At that time, doctors advised us that Vectibix was matched to his "wild-type" KRAS cancer cells, and the treatment should work.

For your information, wild-type KRAS gene makes proteins that regulate cells. If the KRAS gene is mutated, then cancer can be found in the colon, lung, and pancreas. To read more about KRAS wild-type gene, check out the link in the Glossary under KRAS

We were hoping after being on Vectibix for a while, the cancer would all be gone for good. The oncologist advised us that he had several other chemotherapy drugs slated to be approved in the near future that also matched and would be tried if Vectibix failed.

Before Keith could receive infusions of the Vectibix, he first had to have an infusion device installed. This time he had a port-a-cath placed in his chest by the local hospital staff. Here in Keith's own words is his journal entry: *February 18th, 2013, a port-a-cath placed in my chest for follow-up chemo that started the last week of February, Vectibix. This treatment is done every other Monday, and the side effects include skin rashes, which is the hardest thing to manage at this point.*

Doctors ordered a CT scan for March 18, 2013, and again for May 23, 2013, and also for July 17, 2013; all three CT results show the tumor downsizing. A PET scan was ordered, and the insurance company said no, so an MRI was done, which showed the same as the CT scans had shown.

I am now in a wait-and-see mode, still taking Vectibix every other Monday and waiting for the PET scan to be done in February 2014. At this time, my CEA markers are good. The City of Hope shows them in the 1.5 to 1.7 range. The oncologist marker results show 2.3 to 2.6, which is all under the normal of 3.

After much research and speaking with the different physicians and other patients like Keith who had cancer and dealt with cancer markers, we found out that these markers are relevant to the person experiencing cancer. Each is different. Now look at Keith's marker.

One would ask, "What would it be if he had no cancer at all?" Since we don't know because the testing started after the first surgery, we must consider everything. But what we learned through the years was this—To be at three or below was a good thing, meaning the cancer wasn't too active.

Once it started climbing, something was growing. It was pretty low for the longest, considering it was up there in the later years, maybe even 10-13. But, in the end, the marker got to 28-29. Now talk to someone else who has cancer markers, and their markers could be in the thousands. It all depends on the person. It relies on the type of marker also. Keith's marker was CEA, and according to Medlineplus.gov, CEA stands for *carcinoembryonic antigen.*

As you read above, Keith began the new chemotherapy infusions via his new port-a-cath in his upper chest. The port implantation was an extremely rough process for Keith. The doctors at the hospital tried on one side, but it failed, so they had to implant it into the other side. Keith believed the failed attempt on the other side stemmed from the previous infected port in that area.

Afterward, he came home with a swollen neck and upper chest. Poor Keith. He had been through hell with these ports. He had a chest port placed the first year of his chemotherapy treatments only to have it get infected just after they did the first infusion. We prayed that nothing would go wrong with this port.

The good news about this new chemotherapy, Vectibix, was that it did not produce nausea! No nausea at all! The information paper the doctor gave us stated that almost all patients suffer from skin problems ranging from pimples, bumps, rash, dry and cracked skin, plus significant nail problems.

And, all can begin to appear within the first two weeks after the first infusion. Keith was given a small dose of steroids before the chemotherapy infusion on the first go-round. He told me later that it made him feel like his heart was jumping out of his chest for most of the first day. And, when I picked him up, he told me he was starving and famished! This was something new! Usually, he would be nauseous.

By the end of the day, Keith told me he felt weak and shaky when he stood up. He had to slowly stand and stay there collecting himself before proceeding to walk anywhere in the house. Of course, I kept a close eye and arm for him just in case. He also reported a metal taste in his mouth.

As I researched more about Vectibix, I found that it binds to a structure called the epidermal growth factor receptor located on the surface of some cancer cells and normal cells. This therapy is known as a monoclonal antibody and is a man-made version of an immune system protein.

Before the oncologist began this chemotherapy regimen, he consulted with the City of Hope. He ordered a KRAS report on a piece of the biopsied portion of the liver removed in March 2012. They did the report to possibly find better drugs for fighting the cancer in Keith's body.

The days following the Vectibix chemotherapy session on Feb 25, 2013, Keith regained his strength quicker than he had in the past (with other chemotherapies). All was going well until the weekend, when he started getting THE bumps (it appeared like acne but wasn't)—first, just a couple on his nose. Then, every day after that, he gained a few more, and then, suddenly, he had a blast of these ugly, horrible bumps everywhere; in his hair, nose, face, arms, neck, legs, body. Days later they seemed worse because they were bulging, bursting, and bursting.

Keith was in excruciating pain and very uncomfortable. Since we researched everything, we knew the rapidly growing rash wasn't right, so Keith called, and the oncologist prescribed antibiotics to help heal the bumps.

As we have read, everyone is different—some people only experience these bad-grade, two-to-three-bump rashes the first time they have this chemotherapy and only slight rashes later on, but some experience them each chemotherapy infusion.

Keith said they hurt and itched. We were told by the oncologist that ninety-five percent of everyone infused with this chemotherapy experiences the bumps and skin problems.

The oncologist also told us that it was a good sign as it signaled that the drug worked. We prayed that would be true and evident in the next PET scan in June/July.

Another side effect of Vectibix was that Keith's hair became very thick and wiry. Hair began to grow on his body everywhere, including more out-of-control facial hair. On top of the stringy, crazy, growing hair, his face and body were taking a beating with pimples or zits.

As mentioned above, the bumps started small but soon grew into horrible, enormous, painful, pustule pyramids. Quickly I got Keith into our dermatologist's office for a consultation. The doctor prescribed creams and medication. After that, Keith daily slathered on (with my help most of the time) tons of heavy-duty ceramide creams to replenish his skin.

With those same skin-problematic therapies, Keith also suffered greatly from severe toenail problems. The side effects list said that the toenails could possibly lift from the bed of the body and fall off or turn black. Oh My Gosh, or should I say OMG! When I first saw this happening to Keith, I was horrified for him. He took it well, but I knew it upset him to no end. Of course, as usual, I searched for answers to help him through this phase. I found soft foam casings for the toes that allowed Keith to slide them on easily and help keep the nails in place longer.

Keith obviously had to wear good shoes all the time. Going barefoot or wearing sandals would lead to perilous problems if he moved his feet next to something that would move the nail off the bed of the foot.

But on March 13, 2014, a PET scan showed the tumor was still alive in the center and a little around the edge. It was still active! CTs and MRIs completed in May, July, and November 2013 indicated that the tumor was smaller and stable.

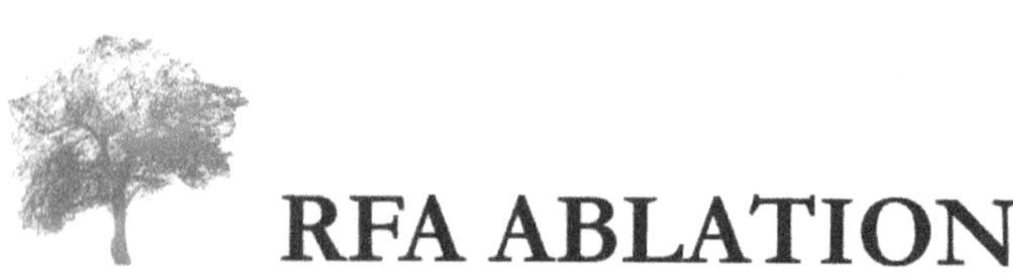

RFA ABLATION

The Y90 spot still was not entirely dead, so the City of Hope planned to do RFA (according to radiologyinfo.org, RFA stands for radiofrequency ablation). Check the link in the Glossary under RFA Ablation.

"**Radiofrequency ablation (RFA)** and microwave ablation (MWA) are treatments that use image guidance to place a needle through the skin into a liver **tumor**. In **RFA**, high-frequency electrical currents are passed through an electrode in the needle, creating a small region of heat." In other words, they went in and cooked the tumor area where they had done the Y90 treatment, leaving the remainder (of what was left) of the liver alone.

April 4, 2014, the City of Hope performed the RFA on the tumor. It took four and a half hours as the doctors wanted to ensure they got it all.

On November 19, 2014, an MRI was done and the test results showed NO NEW cancer, and the RFA-treated tumor decreased in size. Plus, the tumor marker was down to 1.5. Keith continued on the chemotherapy regimen of Vectibix until further notice. Read what Keith said about keeping the cancer under control in February 2015:

Remember I talked about the cancer never being conquered but keeping it under control and knocking it out every time it appeared was the goal of this cancer war. Next, you will notice that the cancer seemed conquered in the liver and now wanted to start a new war in the lungs. The lungs are a frightening place to set up camp. But we were on top of it. Or should I say the City of Hope was on top of it all and taking care of business.

February 18, 2015, came along, and we made our way to the City of Hope for Keith's PET scan and results. Yes, the same day as the tests, we almost always met with the doctor and received the results.

As the doctor read the results, we were almost happy for a quick moment when he told us the tumor that they had ablated in the liver was significantly dead tissue. EXCEPT, and this was when the floor dropped a bit for us; two tiny spots showed activity elsewhere in the liver. The doctor promised to do another ablation and take them out. Wonderful, we thought! Until he continued to give us the not-so-good news that there were three very tiny new spots in both lungs! He told us he had seen them on the last scan but was unsure what they were until today's PET scan. The previous scan was an MRI, which does not show hypermetabolic activity.

Per the City of Hope doctor, the strategy was to consult with Keith's oncologist on the plan for another chemotherapy. Further, Keith's radiologist surgeon would consult with the thoracic specialist at the City of Hope on eradicating the new lung spots.

ZALTRAP WITH COMPTOSAR CHEMOTHERAPIES

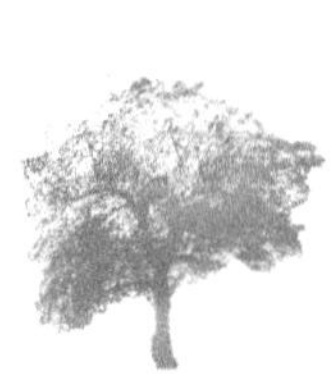

What was next for Keith? Our answers came from both the oncologist and the City of Hope doctor. The plan was to have Keith undergo a six-month-long (every-other-week treatment) intensive chemotherapy to kill the new lung cancer found in February 2015. The primary objective was to go after the lung cancer, and when that decreased or hopefully disappeared, they would go after the spots in the liver. When? The chemotherapy would start on March 23, 2015.

The primary chemotherapy drugs (for a three-hour infusion) were Zaltrap with Comptosar. Keith never received Zaltrap before. The labels list side effects, such as sores in the mouth, hair loss, nausea (they will give Keith anti-nausea meds before his primary chemo treatment each time), and a host of others. Keith would look forward to his skin condition clearing up (since he no longer would be on the Vectibix chemotherapy).

After the others mentioned above, the secondary chemotherapy would be the 5FU via a pump worn by Keith from Monday to Wednesday. We didn't know how this new chemotherapy regimen would affect Keith. In the past, when Keith received chemotherapy from Monday till Wednesday, he usually wasn't feeling too good for the remainder of the week and felt lots better the following week.

We were praying that he would fare well in this new process. Keith needed all the help his angels here on earth, and his angels in Heaven, could muster! I prayed that God and the Universe fight this demon cancer that must be fought and must be killed!

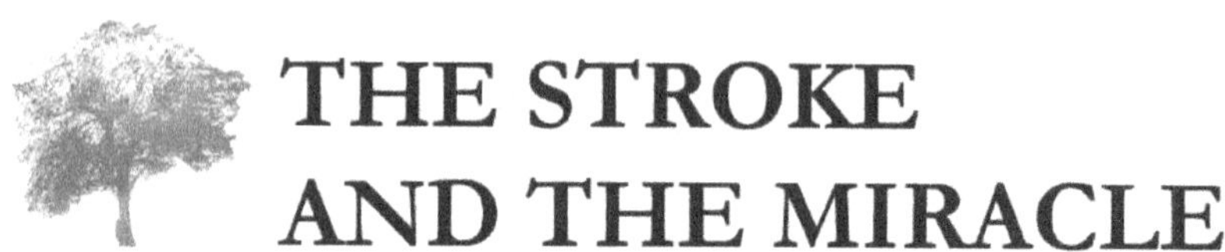

THE STROKE
AND THE MIRACLE

After Keith began the Zaltrap/Comptosar/5FU in late March 2015, he started having issues with spikes in his blood pressure. He was great about taking his blood pressure first thing in the morning, each and every morning. So, he noticed it right away since his blood pressure is usually on the perfect side!

Since quickly getting an appointment with his regular doctor would not happen, we went to the urgent care facility to have Keith examined. Of course, we came with all pertinent information regarding Keith's chemotherapy. The urgent care doctor put Keith on a typical blood pressure pill, which we were diligently monitoring daily. The pill seemed to help control the blood pressure somewhat, up until the first week of July, when, once again, we rushed to the urgent care facility when Keith's blood pressure seemed to be spiking again.

The urgent care doctor that time directed Keith to double the dosage of the blood pressure medication. So this again seemed to help control the blood pressure. But the blood pressure still behaved erratically.

Unfortunately, things turned really bad quickly on the afternoon of July 17, 2015, when Keith was rushed to the hospital, suffering a stroke. Luckily, I was at home with Keith when it happened. If I had been out somewhere and gone for hours, I don't think he would have survived.

It all started on Friday afternoon, and thankfully, we were both in the office. Keith was at his desk facing his bookcases. In the office, we have an entire wall that is built-in bookcases, and then at the bottom left area, there are no drawers underneath to enable sliding a chair under, and there above that, a desk area.

That afternoon I was working at my desk when I noticed Keith was just sitting quietly in front of his laptop computer that he had opened up. It seemed very odd as I did not hear the usual tap-tapping on the keyboard—just silence. I looked over to see if he was looking at a video or reading something. Sometimes he liked to watch videos and would put in earpieces so he wouldn't disturb me. Not that day. He was just sitting there.

I asked him what he was doing, and he responded with something peculiar, so that got my attention, and I got up to look at him. I asked him other questions. His answers were gibberish and didn't make any sense. Since we had been dealing with high blood pressure (due to his chemotherapy) and Keith had just started taking this new double dosage blood pressure pill, I thought I'd better get him back to urgent care (where his doctor prescribed the new medication). So, I gathered him and put him in the car, and drove him right away to Urgent Care.

Along the way, my angels were telling me "Stroke." So, when we arrived inside Urgent Care, I sat Keith down and went to sign him in straightaway, and told the staff, "I think he is having a stroke." They immediately brought him inside, tested him, and called for an ambulance for transport to the hospital. Thankfully, I had taken Keith to Urgent Care in the nearby city. Had I called for the ambulance at our home, they might have taken him to another hospital in the other direction (which I don't recommend). Keith did not have the typical signs of a stroke, such as drooping of the face, not able to raise arms, or trouble walking. But he did not make sense when he talked.

My loudly beating heart rapidly pounded and my own anxiety rose to new extremes as I watched the emergency workers load Keith into the ambulance. I ran to my car to make the drive to the hospital. It was Friday afternoon, with the streets packed with cars going places. When I arrived at the hospital, they had already wheeled Keith back for a CT. When he came back from the CT, as I talked to Keith, a doctor came in, and without any warning, meds, or anything, the doctor started shoving the tracheal intubation tube down Keith's throat. I was aghast!

Keith was still awake, and I thought I would have my own stroke watching that! I was glad Keith couldn't remember that experience because he was struggling and did not look like he was enjoying that at all. Finally, another person came in to help and administered a drug to put him out so they could finish.

Okay, why didn't the meds come first? He was still awake! Then he was out. Not sure that he was out because of the meds, or had he slipped into a coma? When I objected to such treatment, the staff said they had to hurry to get the tube in because they expected him to go into a coma quickly, and his brain might stop his breathing. The news wasn't good. It was downright frightening!

Hemorrhagic bleeding in the brain—That was the CT scan results! The hospital staff checked Keith into the hospital and placed him in the ICU. There he was again, hooked up to all kinds of lines— C-line plus! Tubes everywhere, plus, of course, he was hooked up to a machine that was breathing for him.

This time it wasn't the First Surgical suites, but there was a fold-out bed for me, the waiting wife. I was waiting to know what would become of Keith. So fearful because I had only heard of people dying with this type of stroke. So, there at his side, I stood. Yes, I stood, and I remember this so well.

I stood by his hospital bedside and cried and held his hand for what seemed like hours. The extreme crushing pain of the thought of losing him was almost unmanageable. I continually cried because I felt he was dying and I was losing him. It was a sad situation. I saw what I thought were tears coming from the nurses and doctors when they told me it was dire, alarming, grave. At one point, as I continually bawled, a nurse came in and asked if I had anyone to be with me. I guess I looked like I needed to be cared for as well.

At one point, I remembered that we had prayer groups. I got on my cell phone and started writing an email to the prayer group requesting big prayers for Keith and letting them know what happened. Our priest wrote back quickly and presented that he was praying. Soon, I received many offering prayers. I prayed also. I prayed harder than ever before, asking God to heal Keith and assist the doctors. And I requested the intercession of the saints for healing help. It was a desperate time, and we needed everyone's help! Save my husband, please, was my plea!

After praying, I prayed more at his bedside, standing vigil there for hours on end until I could no longer stand. I think I was not even thinking about feeling my legs until hours later when I suddenly felt my legs were very heavy. That feeling pushed me to sit on the chair I pushed next to the end of Keith's bed. There was too much equipment that kept me from sitting next to Keith's head area. It was hard to leave his side, but my legs would no longer hold me up. I moved from the chair finally and opened the fold-out bed, placed sheets, lay down, covered up, and cried and prayed more. I never slept, but I closed my eyes and rested my weary body.

The nurses scurried in to check on Keith and put in new IV bags and meds as needed. They kept track of his status from their stations for most of the time. Many times, the alarms would go on, and I would find a nurse to help. One nurse taught me how to turn off the noise-making machine (after making sure they know of the alarm), thinking it might wake Keith up. But, wait a minute, we need to wake him up! Maybe Not YET?

At some point, a doctor came in, and I think he said he was the doctor for the floor that night, and he wanted to talk about palliative care. Meaning "this is IT" kind of care. It got me angry. It could be I was in my "fight it" mode, and it may have been that I was overly tired and worn through and through, but don't mess with me was where I was. So, my response to the doctor was that he should concentrate on helping my husband wake up and be well and out of this situation and find a doctor to resolve the hemorrhaging. But don't talk to me about palliative care as we have not given up! Period. The doctor just walked away. He couldn't take me, and I couldn't take him that night. We were not ready to give up!

Before this time, they had taken Keith down for an MRI of the brain. Moving him was no simple feat for someone who was on a ventilator. They had to hook up a special long hose to place the ventilator machine outside the MRI room's door while they did the MRI testing. Other devices could not be near the MRI machine while it was running. Once he got back in the room, they removed the super-duper long attachment.

After the MRI, I kept thinking a doctor or someone would come and let me know the MRI results, but no one did. I asked the nurse, and she said they would come to me when they could. It was a weekend and things did not work fast at the hospital on weekends.

Angel?

MUCH LATER IN THE NIGHT, it happened. It could have been around midnight, or one a.m. It was very late. Much of the hallways and areas were primarily quiet and more dimly lit. I wanted to believe the nurses and staff were sitting there watching all the patient's machines and readings on the computers.

I was once again standing with Keith by the side of his bed. I wasn't crying. I was all cried out. I stood facing the door and the desks at ICU central. I could see a person walking seemingly toward our room. This person stood reasonably tall, was thin, and wore a brilliant white outfit. As he came into view, I could see his clothing was unlike hospital staff clothing, such as doctors' usual white coats. For the life of me, I thought I saw an angel!

I swear he glowed as he walked through the darkened corridor. Dressed in extremely fine white, he continued to our room. Then I saw him more clearly. He wore a beautiful delicate white fez hat with a glimmering white tassel streaming down from the top. A white, perfect, impeccable linen, extremely long shirt, and impeccably sharp white pants made up the rest of his attire. And, his face I will never forget.

One name came to my mush of a mind instantly: Omar Sharif. Yes, he looked like the Egyptian actor, who played Sherif Ali on the Laurence of Arabia movie, with a gorgeous Fez hat! Angelic? Oh yes! And did I say he glowed? Perhaps his white was so white, and it was so dark everywhere, his outfit glowed? I don't know. But even today, I still believe I saw an angel and perhaps a miracle. As I stood by Keith's bed totally astounded, the man approached and reached across the bed and extended his hand to me. I shook his hand, still gazing and transfixed as to what and who I was seeing. I don't recall him telling me his name. I only remember that he told me that he just looked at the MRI, and he said, "Your husband will be fine. The bleed is small, and he will make a full recovery." Wow, can you imagine my thoughts then? Rejoicing, or did I hear that right? I asked, "He will recover?" and he responded, "Yes!" Astounded, I watched as he turned around and disappeared back into the darkened corridor once again.

After that, I began to fight more to get Keith's condition changed so that he could come back to us. I knew the longer he was on the ventilator, the more problems he could have, and recovery could be hampered or fail altogether. With that news, I went back to lie down in the bed and rested. I was up and down the rest of the night, but I wasn't crying any longer. I had new hope that Keith would survive.

The next day was a long one. One doctor after another came in to see Keith. First, there was the hospitalist and plenty of nurses streaming in. Then, the respiratory crew came to help keep Keith's airways clear. The doctors kept trying to wean Keith off of his meds that kept him in the coma. But every time they did, Keith went into flailing mode like he was having an attack of some sort. They were giving him propofol, and its withdrawal effects were crazy. I was getting exasperated and felt that other drugs needed to be used instead of propofol. What if they changed the propofol to something else? Finally, a Latina doctor came on duty. She was feisty like me, and we almost locked heads, but she finally understood what I was asking of her. That there should be another way. And finally, that doctor changed Keith's meds. The respiratory therapist was there.

Thirty minutes after the nurse administered the new meds to Keith, I saw Keith's arms moving. I rushed to his side to help. Just in case, he began a fit as he had done before when he tried to dislodge the tube from his throat. His hands were tied down, but he could still move a lot. I saw his eyes open wide and follow me as I approached him. Then I noticed his tied-down hands trying to motion me to remove the restraints. He was distraught because he could not move, but he was not flailing uncontrollably (as before)!

The therapist, who still stood there by him, looked at him and then me, and I asked Keith if he could see me, and he nodded "yes." Wow, he was back! He understood what I said! He still had the ventilator hooked up and breathing for him with the tube down his throat, so he could not speak.

But he did point to it calmly, motioning what was this and what happened. Meanwhile, I called the nurse to report to the doctor what had happened. It was a miracle. He seemed lucid, calm, and understanding. The doctor came in and exclaimed, "I have never seen this happen before!" So, see, it was a miracle. The respiratory therapist also said she had not witnessed a recovery like that either.

The doctor wanted to leave the ventilator on him longer and even talked about leaving it overnight, thinking if he reverted back to a coma, they would have to insert it again and risk re-insertion problems. I fought that since I knew Keith would not want that in him that long. It was killing me, so he must have been tortured by the ventilator intubation. Thankfully, the doctor finally relented because the respiratory therapist was still there.

The therapist would assist by weaning Keith slowly from the ventilator and make sure Keith could breathe independently for a while before unhooking and removing the ventilator completely. Little by little, the respiratory therapist and nurse worked until finely the ventilator was removed entirely. What a relief that was for him and me! Whew! Next, Keith had to try to talk—a little at a time. The nurses and doctors came in asking and testing his cognitive situation. The first thing I noticed was he had trouble reading. He was finally able to eat. So, he could order breakfast for the following morning. I handed him the menu but he said he couldn't read the words on the menu.

That night, he had all liquid to make sure he could swallow okay after having that tube down his throat. It seemed like other faculties were there. After a time, they got him to sit on the side of the bed with more tests. He was then standing up. He could stand and be steady also. And, take steps, yes, he did that fine. After all the tests, it appeared that the only problem was his vision. Keith could not read.

Later in the evening, when it was all quiet (well, relatively quiet considering it is never tranquil in a hospital) and the hallways dimly lit, our angel arrived again. I swear it was that kind man from the night before who said Keith would survive his stroke! But this time, the man wore a gorgeous, long, gold jacket, white linen pants, and a glimmering gold fez hat with a gorgeous gold tassel hanging from the top of the hat. And that time, my husband was awake! He came to Keith's bedside, shook Keith's hand, and introduced himself. To this day, I still can't remember his name. I just think of Omar Sharif.

The doctor articulated that the bleed happened around the optical nerve, which was the reason for the reading problems. He told us that the situation would resolve itself over time with therapist home visits ordered for the next four months—The therapy sessions indeed helped Keith with his optical problems.

The stately dressed doctor concluded the talk again, adding that Keith would make a full recovery and be fine. While he was in the room with us, a nurse came in, and she mentioned something about Keith meeting his neurologist for the first time. The doctor was greatly offended and quickly whipped his head in her direction and expressed to the nurse, in no uncertain terms, that he was NOT a neurologist but a neurosurgeon. A significant difference, he advised the nurse. The nurse quickly left the room, figuring she must make herself scarce quickly.

He was nice to Keith and me, and in the end, I got up the nerve to ask him if people ever mistook him for a movie star? He smiled and laughed (but did not answer my question) and then said goodbye. We never saw him again. After a month, Keith had a follow-up meeting with a regular neurologist recommended by the hospital.

On August 21, 2015, Keith had an MRI of his head to check on the hematoma. The doctor told us the results were good. The hematoma (bleeding area) was stable, with no new bleeding or CVAs (cerebrovascular accident) reported. The hematoma is in the late subacute stage. Basically, here are the different stages for strokes—Hyperacute (1 day from stroke), Acute (1-3 days), early subacute (3-7 days), late subacute (7-14 days), chronic (14-28 days).

To understand more about MRI stroke staging, go to the interesting site for more detail that is listed in the Glossary under MRI Stroke Staging.

Meanwhile, Keith could go from his recuperating, slow-turtle mode to semi-moderate mode with this good news. The neurologist wanted to see the hematoma decrease in size a lot before Keith could go back to full "SWING" mode. We were okay with this, given what could have been. Keith's other energy-zapping came from the many meds he received. We hoped these meds would be decreased in time, which would help him regain even more strength and endurance. I created elaborate spreadsheets to keep track of the umpteen pills Keith had to take each day.

That neurologist scheduled an MRI for three months later. After the follow-up MRI, and subsequent neurologist appointment, there was further proof of a miracle. The neurologist told us that the MRI did not show that Keith ever had a stroke, hemorrhagic, or any other type of stroke event ever at all!

He went on to say that hemorrhagic strokes usually show a mass that gets smaller with time (usually a few years) and always show a scar or evidence. The neurologist said he knew the radiologist who wrote the MRI results and completely trusted his judgment. Further, he said that if the MRI had been done elsewhere, he would question it.

There was no evidence the stroke ever happened! Stroke of a Miracle! Keith was in a coma for over thirty hours and survived.

Needless to say, no more Zaltrap. Yes, we confirmed that Zaltrap could cause strokes. The side effects of all the chemotherapies were staggering. Keith didn't start back on chemotherapy until October. And it did not include Zaltrap.

<u>Amazing Keith continued to recover!</u> Yes, he went home to recuperate. After receiving yet another script for steroids, Keith felt better. The steroids helped the inflammation in his brain (he had experienced constant, never-ending headaches since his release from the hospital). His blood pressure was also back to normal (like before the chemotherapy started in March with the Zaltrap).

Thankfully, a trip to the ophthalmologist on July 27, 2015 (a couple weeks after the stroke), revealed NO permanent stroke damage to his optical region. However, he was still experiencing fuzzy vision and reading difficulties (which other doctors indicated should dissipate with time from the bleeding and assimilate in the body). Meanwhile, he underwent speech therapy to help the process of relearning/resyncing the damaged area of the brain. Go to the Glossary under Stroke to find more information.

Research revealed that sixty-four percent of people suffering hemorrhagic/intracranial strokes die, and among the remaining survivors, only ten percent survive without any impairments. We still considered the recovery a Miracle for Keith. Of course, we thanked God for all blessings continuously bestowed upon Keith's healing.

But what about chemotherapy? The oncologist planned to start Keith on chemotherapy in mid-September. The plan was to use a drug in the same family as his previous chemotherapy, which affected his skin and hair. Plus, adding another previous drug that Keith had received that did not influence his blood pressure or bleeding in the body. Something interesting the oncologist said about the stroke and cancer—he said that he often saw the cancer frozen in time and not progressing because the body's fighting machines are in full fight mode during a major bodily event such as a stroke. We were afraid that since he had not had chemotherapy for a long time, the cancer would have been growing faster. Not usually the case, the oncologist told us.

Finally, months after the July stroke, and of course, the stoppage of chemotherapy, a PET scan was completed September 30, 2015, on Keith (from the neck down). The results were fascinating to us! IT SHOWED NO CANCER ACTIVITY IN KEITH'S LIVER!!!! YEAH!!!!

Thankfully, regarding the cancer nodes in the lungs, the test results showed a miniscule increase in size. We remembered viewing both the March and September scan results with the doctor. The March PET scan showed the liver cancer mass lit up with hypermetabolic activity, indicating the cancer cells were alive. The September scan showed nothing lit up at all. This was very encouraging! The doctors said it meant the chemotherapies worked.

Meanwhile, after Keith had an MRI on his head on October 15, 2015, and doctors cleared him, chemotherapy started again on October 19, 2015. He had had no chemotherapy since June 14, 2015.

The new regimen did NOT include the drug Zaltrap, which the oncologist believed was the culprit that brought on the hemorrhagic brain bleed. Part of the new chemotherapy would be back to the maintenance type of chemotherapy (Erbitux), affecting Keith's skin and hair. In the past, when Keith received this type of chemotherapy, he would feel good the next day. The oncologist added additional chemotherapy, Camptosar. Keith had been given this drug before but usually in addition to other chemotherapy drugs. So, we hoped that it would not provide him with long-term side effects.

On July 27, 2016 (a year after the stroke), an MRI and CT scan of the abdomen and chest with contrast showed that all tumors were smaller and shrinking in size. As per the radiologist doctor at the City of Hope, it was time to go after the tumors in the lungs and take them out. The City of Hope offered several options—RFA (radiofrequency ablation) or radiation.

Since we wanted a greater understanding of the different options available, we received a referral to a local radiologist. We made an appointment (which took a lot of doing and a lot of time till the appointment). Once at the meeting, both Keith and I quickly formed an immediate opinion. Neither of us wanted radiation to be part of the plan of action to take out the lung cancer.

It seemed to us that there was a whole gamut of things that could possibly go wrong while being treated by radiation. And many resulting problems would have been long-term ramifications. Radiation long-term side effects would leave permanent issues and scars. And radiation on the lungs being near so many exceedingly vital organs was a terrifying thought to both of us. But wait. There was another way.

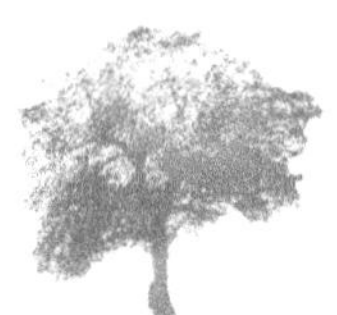

CRYOABLATION

s it turned out, God had another plan for us to save Keith once
more! The radiologist surgeon at the City of Hope advised he
would perform a cryoablation on the lung lesions. So glad we decided
on the radiologist surgeon to perform the cryoablation in Keith's
lung. Since this was new to us, we were also very apprehensive, but
we knew it had to be done. It was an all-day procedure, performed
through the skin, piercing into the lung, starting early morning and
lasting to the evening.

This information about cryoablation is from Mayoclinic.org:
"Cryoablation for cancer is a treatment to kill cancer cells with
extreme cold. A thin, wand-like needle (cryoprobe) is inserted
through your skin and directly into the cancerous tumor during
cryoablation. Gas is pumped into the cryoprobe to freeze the tissue.
Then the tissue is allowed to thaw. The freezing and thawing process
is repeated several times during the same treatment session." Check
out the Glossary for an informative link.

So, there I sat, in the waiting area again, and I felt that I was on
the verge of weeping for some reason. My mind went briefly back to

my feelings of the previous July when I almost lost Keith. But I told myself everything would be okay, because the City of Hope took great care of Keith. Nevertheless, I sat on pins and needles, nervously waiting for the surgery to be over.

Pneumothorax

ONCE KEITH WAS IN THE recovery area, they ushered me back there to be with him. The doctor appeared to tell of good coverage of the lesion on the left lung (they can only do one lung at a time) and that Keith would be there a while since there was a pneumothorax because they had to puncture the lung to get in there with the equipment. I quickly studied up on this new word–Pneumothorax. From Mayoclinic.org, they explain: "A **pneumothorax** occurs when air leaks into the space between your lung and chest wall. This air pushes on the outside of your lung and makes it collapse. **Pneumothorax** can be a complete lung collapse or a collapse of only a portion of the lung." Check out the link in the Glossary under Pneumothorax.

Thankfully, Keith only had a partial collapse. They kept giving him oxygen and bringing in the X-ray equipment and checking until they finally announced the pneumothorax had all but closed up. Then they released Keith, and I drove us home. I might add that driving to and from the City of Hope has never been a joy of mine. We were usually driving in at least one direction in heavy traffic. But getting released after rush hour was big, and we thankfully sailed home quickly.

We were much concerned about venturing into the cryoablation of the lung area. Before the surgery, I researched as I usually did to learn all I could. We learned that the lesions were in the bronchopleural. We also learned what to look for afterward, such as hemoptysis, coughing up blood from the lungs—thanking God that did not happen.

Thoracentesis

WE ALSO LEARNED ABOUT ANOTHER problem that could have happened (and thankfully didn't): hemothorax, an accumulation of blood and fluid in the pleural cavity. Another scary term came up: thoracentesis, to remove excess fluid in the space between the lungs and chest wall in treating pleural effusions (excess fluid in the pleural space) and thanking God once again that Keith did not experience any of these complications or problems.

On November 11, 2016, another cryoablation was performed on Keith's other lung by the radiologist surgeon of City of Hope. This time the pneumothorax healed quickly and did not show on the x-rays with Keith released in record time.

It is now January 2017, and we had a scary ER (emergency at the hospital) visit for Keith. Keith wrote: *Taken to ER at the hospital for a bowel blockage. Surgery was immediately on the ER doctor's mind. I referred them to my liver surgeon, who stopped any talk of another surgery. My bowel was twisted, and I have no food or water with an NG tube in my nose.*

Keith began having issues with his bowels at home, and they seized up and were not working at all. We thought it was because of steak he had eaten the night before since we rarely ate beef. But we never really found out the real reason for the paralyzed colon.

Because a section of Keith's colon had a quirk in it (as we were to find out), the colon began to twist on itself in that area and became paralyzed. As I recall, this was the section where they had rejoined Keith's colon after the primary initial bowel resection at the time the doctors discovered the cancer.

We rarely had steak or beef after that because this paralyzed colon problem was just so scary. Keith was in the hospital for three days, most of it without food or water and with the nasty nasal tube down his nose to his stomach to drain the bile out.

They had to do that until his colon started working again. Again, they put him through taking the contrast while shooting pictures of his colon, and it ended up un-paralyzing his colon so that it was back working again.

I find it interesting to note that just six days earlier, on January 11, 2017, Keith had gone to the dentist's office, where he had to have a fractured tooth extracted. He suffered fractured teeth often due to the chemotherapy treatments.

Now, what I find thought-provoking, and I question whether there was a correlation. A correlation between Keith receiving a tooth extraction plus socket preservation technique insertion including cow bone to strengthen the area done on January 11, 2017, and his intestines/colon seizing up January 17, 2017? Makes a person wonder if bacteria floated its way down to the intestine from the mouth and set up a bad situation in Keith's intestine/colon flora and helped cause the paralyzed body part? We did ask various doctors and they did tell us that they had seen dental work problems cause other body repercussions. Thereafter, we carefully watched when dental work was performed.

February 1, 2017, we were at City of Hope again for blood work, CT, and MRI of the abdomen and chest with contrast. The results showed there was new growth in the liver near the crown. Yikes! It had been a long time since new growth anywhere. August 2017 MRI and CT test results show no change.

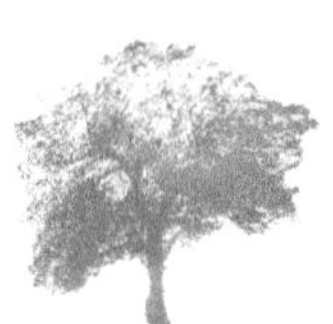

VALENTINE FUN

Upon learning the test results (February 1st) about the new growth (in the liver) stressed both Keith and me. So, we set off to extinguish those anxieties in a fashion that we have become accustomed to.

In February 2017, Keith surprised me by booking a night for a Valentine's celebration at the famed Madonna Inn in San Luis Obispo. We had been there before (Madonna Inn) and loved it because they offered a lovely dance floor and dancing nearly every night. For this time, Keith booked the Edelweiss Room for our stay. This particular weekend was special because of the surprise and also because we got a specific room with a patio overlooking the green pasture for the horses. We spent hours watching the white horse and old-fashioned white carriage pick up valentine's guests for a ride. We enjoyed watching more than participating. Later on, we would find our way to the Inn's fine dining opulent restaurant and once again pretend we were back in the day when huge booths and tables with real tablecloths and fine China in restaurants were in fashion. After an abalone dinner (for me, lobster for Keith), the dancing began. We danced as much as Keith could handle, and then we retired.

Mary's Mother Passes

IN AUGUST 2017, my mother ended up in the hospital. It was a complete surprise because she had been doing great. At eighty-eight years, she still lived at home but used a walker (because of a hip problem). Otherwise, her health had been good for a while.

Then we got a call to see her at the hospital. Upon our arrival, she announced, "I am finished!" That was a shocker, and I asked her what she meant by that statement. She told us that she had lived to raise her great-grandson, and now that he had graduated high school, Mom was finished with that project and ready to leave life.

My mother raised her great-grandson all of his life. She had raised his mother also. He is the grandson of my brother, who passed away resulting from a motorcycle accident back in 1978. You see, my brother had just married a few months before his death, and his wife was pregnant with the great-grandson's mother. My brother's death messed up his wife, driving her to turn to drugs. Once she gave birth, it was evident that she could not properly care for the baby, and my mother (and father) gained authority and raised the great-grandson's mother and subsequently the great-grandson himself.

Not long after the hospital stay I mentioned above, Mom went into hospice care in a private care home. And, by mid-October 2017, she was gone. Losing her so quickly was a real shocker since my mom had always been the strongest person I knew before Keith.

After Mom died, we had to sell her property. This left the great-grandson alone. As it turned out, the great-grandson had nowhere to go. Keith and I had to take him in; otherwise, he would be spending his life on the streets. You see, the great-grandson had several problems that kept him from fending for himself—He was autistic and had other developmental issues.

As soon as we got the great-grandson (my great-nephew) home

to live with us, we saw lots more problems than we might be able to handle. Therefore, I sought help for my great-nephew from every avenue possible. Finally, we found a service for people with disabilities such as autism, and significant support began to materialize for my great-nephew and us.

Meanwhile, for the first time ever, my great-nephew had a strong man to help support him—Keith. Keith meant a lot to him. He even wrote in a greeting card to Keith that he was his savior in saving him from the cruel world. Keith talked with him and helped him as much as he could during Keith's time dealing with cancer. Keith was always a giving person, no matter how he felt.

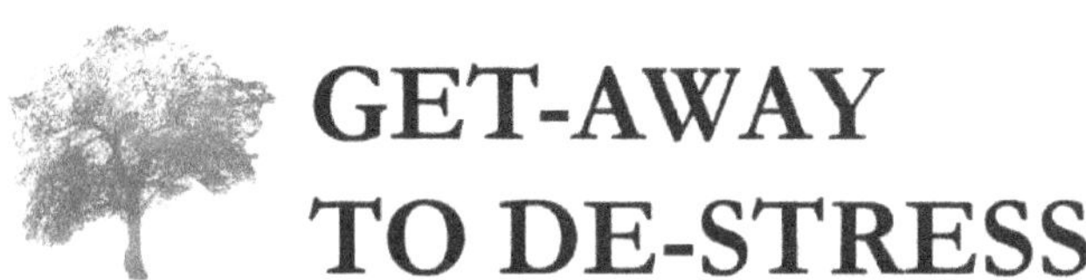

GET-AWAY TO DE-STRESS

It is interesting to note that sometimes our time away from it all was figured out and planned ahead of time. In this case, these next two trips had been pre-planned and so very needed. But we had not designed to be saying goodbye to my mother and getting ready to take on a whole new responsibility in the midst of our trips.

Keith and I planned a trip along with Keith's life-long friend and his wife for the first week of September, 2017. It was to be Keith's and his life-long friend's fiftieth friendship anniversary trip. The excursion would begin in Oregon and trail down thru the magnificent coastal Redwoods of California. As we had done throughout the cancer journey, we designed the chemotherapy around the trip and even planned a trip back to Northern California to see Keith's other long-time friend and wife at Lake Almanor. We made both of these one-week trips with just a week in between. And, yes, my mother was placed in hospice care in the midst of our travels. I had thought of staying at home to see about my mother but Keith told me that my mother would want me to go and get away from it all. Of course, I did not want to be away from my dear Keith either.

As I think I've indicated before, we planned trips to give us something to look forward to instead of always looking to the subsequent treatment, surgery, or test.

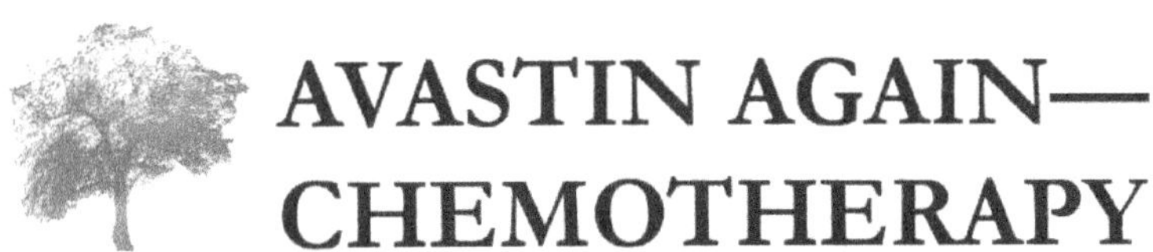

AVASTIN AGAIN—
CHEMOTHERAPY

In February 2018, a CT and MRI showed an increase in the size of the left upper lobe nodule and the development of new pulmonary nodules.

Time for yet another chemotherapy. It was thought that the Erbitux's effects were beginning to wane. So, the oncologist decided it was time for another try at a chemotherapy Keith had at the beginning of his cancer journey—Avastin. It had helped Keith back then and rid the cancer totally for a while.

March 26, 2018, Keith started on the new chemotherapy regimen—Avastin, Leucovorin, and 5FU (the pump).

But before Keith began his new chemotherapy, we figured out how Keith's stamina was holding up and planned a de-stressing vacation. We found out our grandchildren in Texas had a spring break coming up, and we jumped at the chance to visit with them and the family.

Instead of sitting at home worrying about the new developments in the cancer area, we jumped in the pool with the grandchildren and enjoyed their company.

The next leg of our almost two-week vacation we spent in sunny Florida. Where we visited Orlando's parks and Kennedy Space Center. The entire time Keith experienced a great deal of energy. He was able to walk thru the parks at length and with ease. I took more photos of Keith smiling ear to ear! He enjoyed himself so much that I did not want to speak about the nag—Cancer. And, the upcoming new chemotherapy regimen on March 26, 2018.

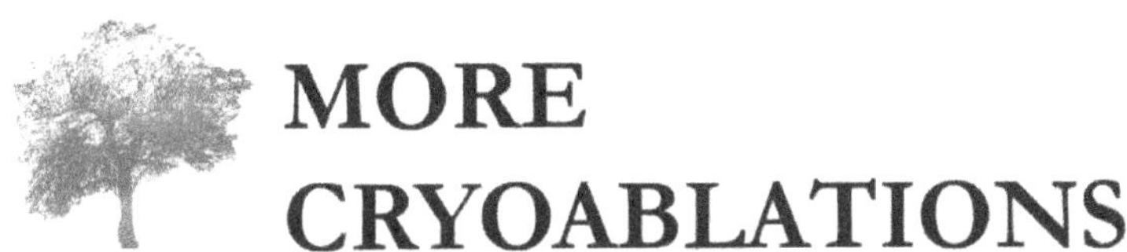

MORE CRYOABLATIONS

On June 21, 2018, we were at the City of Hope for two more cryoablations. One on the right lung and the other at the top of the liver. The radiologist surgeon advised us that he did both cryoablations with one hundred percent coverage.

July 5, 2018, we were back to the City of Hope for the cryoablation in the left lung. The insertion point was at the nipple (ouch) to reach the lung tumor.

Without dancing in the midst of chemotherapy, tests and cryoablations and our small and large get-aways, it would have been more difficult to get through Keith's cancer journey.

In July of 2018 we were lucky enough to attend an incredible concert at the brilliant Disney Hall. We learned early on to book a seat on the terrace levels just above the orchestra on the violin side. That way, we could see everything happening on the left side of the orchestra. We enjoyed being in the over-watching area immensely! I had been a violinist in the school orchestras in my young years.

Two months later in September, an event Keith and I began a few years in the past and tried to make it each year since, was the Cruising for a Cure classic car show at the Orange County raceway. The only classic car show we know where we could sit down, and the classic cars would cruise past us while bands played nearby.

Later in September, another fun time getaway down in San Diego—Miramar Airshow with the Blue Angels. In years past, we attended, but this would be the ultimate experience because we were sitting smack dab at center line. Everything happened right there in front of us like nothing before. Keith was in ecstasy! We stayed overnight at a hotel just across from the Marine base, got up early, and got our seats quickly saved under the tents at our reserved area. Great idea! Back when I attended air shows in the 80's we came with umbrellas and chairs and coolers, walking for miles to sit and then walking for miles to see all the static show items (planes and such). That September day, we arrived and for the day, we had our seats under the tents all ready for us. We were supplied our morning muffins or Danish (it was just after 8 am) and drinks, then, later on, a full-on banquet, hot buffet meal was served with drinks. It was hot and sunny, but as the day moved along, the clouds appeared to make our videos and photos of the jets, planes, helicopters, parachuters extra special. It was the most memorable day Keith talked about a long time.

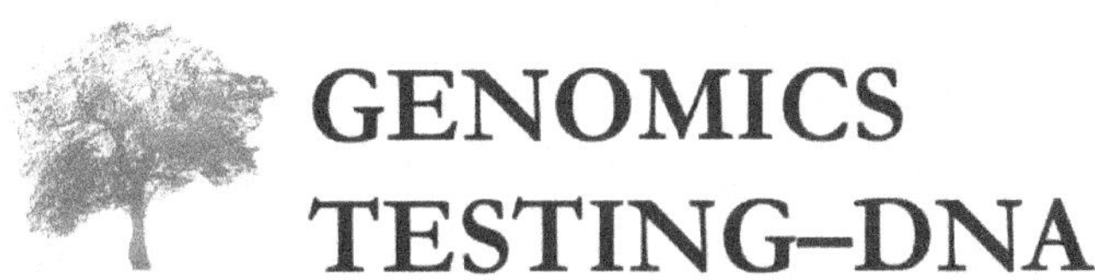

GENOMICS TESTING–DNA

November 7, 2018, NEO Genomics testing was ordered by the City of Hope on the tissue of 2012. The tissue of 2012 was back when Keith had the resection of half his liver done by the hospital. At that time, they saved specimens and froze them. The City of Hope needed to know more about the cancer found in 2012. Six years later, DNA had become a much bigger help fighting health problems.

After all that talk about DNA and Genomics testing, we had to seek some happy times. Keith was always searching for opportunities to place his mind into another realm and help with the positive thoughts and feelings.

Later in November, Keith, my great-nephew, and I, along with a couple of friends, attended the awe-inspiring seventy-fifth-year anniversary celebration of the restaurant chain In-N-Out held at the Pomona raceway.

We witnessed iconic Top Fuel and other race cars speeding down the famed race track where the Winter Nationals of drag racing is held each year. Keith was happy because his favorite food (sans fries), In-N-Out, was served in abundance. Keith and I were beyond delighted to be able to put in the earplugs and climb onto the spectator stands. We jumped up at the thrill as we watched and felt the rip-roaring, ground rumbling, body pulsating Top Fuel dragsters, Funny Cars, and classic cars race down the one-thousand-foot track (it used to be a quarter-mile track).

Keith loved to tell about his racing days when he took his own souped-up cars to the historic Lions Drag Strip in Wilmington, California, and raced often. I know I was there. I must have seen him. But I didn't know him back then. Both Keith and I had a love of super-fast funny cars, dragsters, classic cars, and the racetrack.

On February 13, 2019, we were back at the City of Hope, this time for a CT and follow-up with the doctor. He told us everything was stable. Mind you, this is only a CT and did not show hypermetabolic activity like a PET scan does. The insurance does not allow but one PET scan a year.

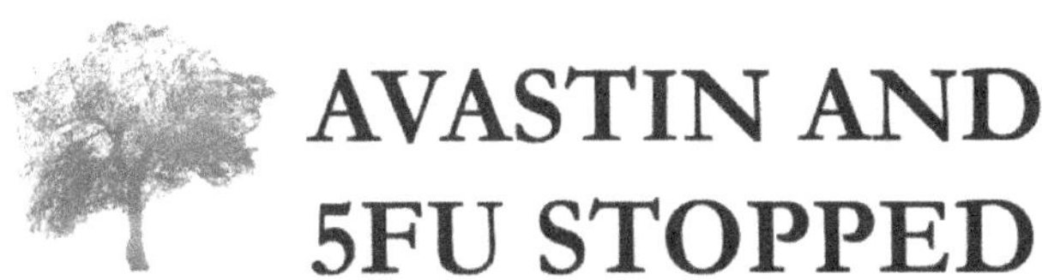 AVASTIN AND 5FU STOPPED

It was April 2019 and Keith was still receiving the chemotherapy protocol we spoke about in March 2018—Avastin, Leucovorin, and 5FU (the pump). Just so you know, while Keith was on Avastin, etc., he could not receive any surgical procedures. Each time doctors scheduled surgery for Keith, he had to be off the chemotherapy for at least four weeks before and after any surgical procedures. We were greatly worried that this loss of chemotherapy time would promote new cancer growth.

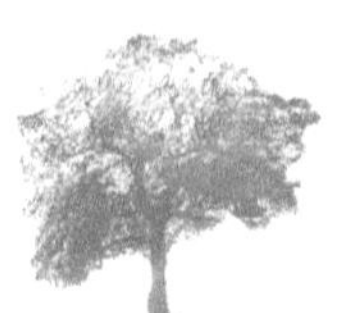

GENOMIC TESTING

It was May 15, 2019, and we were back at the City of Hope for a CT and MRI. Thankfully, we always received our results the same day as the tests. The doctor revealed that the liver tumor (that they previously ablated) showed growth. But doctors needed a PET scan to confirm what they suspected.

Meantime they planned a biopsy of the current liver cancer lesion on May 24, 2019, so that they could send that biopsy to pathology and genomics testing to possibly find a new chemotherapy regimen (since the Avastin, etc. protocol stopped being effective). The fear was that the cancer had evolved over the years. So, the doctors thought procuring a biopsy of a current bit of cancer within Keith could bring new information on how to treat him.

The City of Hope ran two genomics tests on this new biopsy. To our great surprise, the first test showed HER2 negative, and the second tested HER2 positive. Since they were contradictory, City of Hope sent a biopsy sample directly to Genentech, the company known for more than thirty years researching and testing, finding the HER2 gene, and producing chemotherapy that fights cancer (mainly breast) caused by hyperactivity in the HER2 gene.

The report from Genentech showed HER2 positive and recommended Herceptin and Perjeta as therapeutic drugs.

It was June 27, 2019, and Keith was back at the City of Hope again for another cryoablation in the liver and two RFAs also in the liver. My brother was with him that time since I was not in town. I was distraught because I was not there with Keith. All those years I had always been there with him every moment of the way never wanting to leave his side for anything. But that appointment was last-minute and I couldn't get back in town until that evening.

Thank goodness for my great brother. I arrived later in the evening to find Keith doing well and resting from the ordeal that day. Keith told me the doctor advised that everything went well, and that he was able to take care of all the lesions they planned to take out of commission. I would find out later on that Keith didn't quite hear everything correctly and that there was one spot the doctor could not touch because it was much too near an artery.

Trying to still find a good answer on the protocol for saving Keith, on July 15, 2019, we met with a doctor in a medical institute that was so secretive that I could not reveal the name. They are researchers for cancer, so of course, we were interested in what the doctor had to say.

This medical research place was so secretive that the front desk personnel scanned our identification. We had to wear arm bracelets and be escorted everywhere in the building at all times. We were instructed not to take out our cell phones for any reason while in the building. Wow!

The doctor at the institute there was greatly interested in helping Keith. He had a particular blood plasma test run that he said would show everything needed to know about his cancer. Amazing! I thought to myself, "Why don't all medical organizations have this test?"

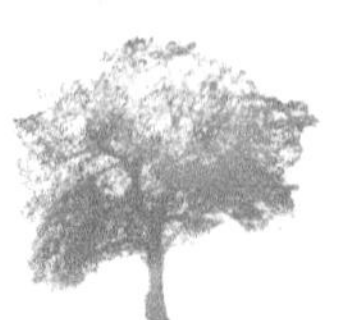

HER2 AND BRCA2

From this plasma test, on July 24, 2019, we received a written report that showed alterations to Keith's DNA after being born (not passed onto any children). Keith's BRCA2 gene was 5.9 percent, and the HER2 (ERBB2) was amplified medium double positive. This news meant that something altered his DNA after Keith was born. Recall back when I told the story of watching the *Brockovich* movie and chromium poisoning? This confirmed what we had suspected— something had altered Keith's DNA and a causal factor in the creation of the cancer.

Now I should tell you what my research found on these two genes I mentioned in the previous paragraph. You see, the HER2 and BRCA2 genes are cancer-fighting genes. They usually work for our protection to keep cancer away. However, when these genes go into hyperactivity metabolically, they turn into cancer-producing cells instead. Read more about it at the CDC link listed in our Glossary.

PERJETA AND HERCEPTIN

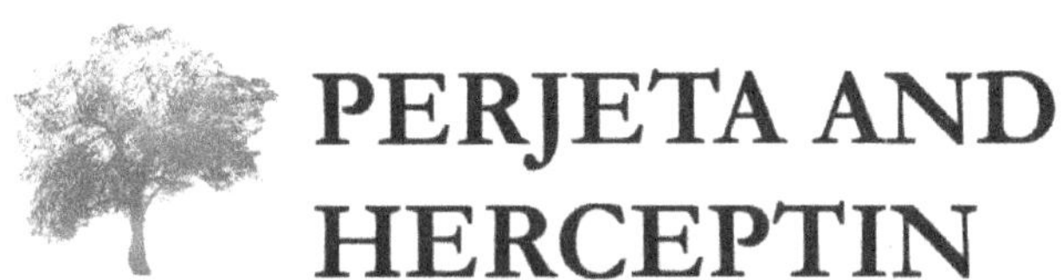

The doctor from the medical research facility recommended the same therapies as the City of Hope and Genentech recommended—Herceptin and Perjeta. He also advised adding Avastin back into the mix along with 5FU. He also advised echocardiograms to be performed every three months because Perjeta's side effects could mess with the heart.

I found more information from the Perjeta website. I found that "too much Her2" "causes cells to grow and divide rapidly," thus producing cancer cells. You see, HER2 ("human epidermal growth factor receptor 2") contains "receptors found on the surface of cells." And, the "job is to tell it to grow and divide." Read more in a link listed in the Glossary under Perjeta.:

Keith's oncologist was hesitant to shove all those chemicals on Keith too quickly. So, the strategy was to start with the infusions of the Herceptin and Perjeta every three weeks. Then, later begin introducing the Avastin and 5FU infusions on weeks other than when the Herceptin and Perjeta got infused.

As it turned out, the Herceptin and Perjeta infusions began September 8, 2019, and the Avastin/5FU combination didn't start until two days before Christmas. Keith's oncologist was always watching out for Keith and protecting him. Keith had bleeding in November that absolutely stalled the Avastin (it can cause bleeding), but Keith hadn't even started on it yet!

Before the Perjeta and Herceptin started, we were at the City of Hope for Keith's MRI on August 7, 2019. The results were scary! They showed three small new spots in the liver, with one running along the seam of the lobe where they had done the resection. And one close to the portal artery they had tried to ablate in June 2019 but failed. The doctor at the City of Hope said he would contact the oncologist to make sure Keith was on maintenance chemotherapy right away since he had not been on anything since May 2019.

As mentioned above, Keith began receiving treatments with the new regimen of drugs, Herceptin and Perjeta, on September 8, 2019. As soon as I brought Keith home after those infusions, Keith told me he was experiencing chills. I could see him shiver like crazy and wrapped him up, then called the oncologist nurse to report Keith's condition.

The nurse advised that Keith needed to take Benadryl to relieve the reaction. Benadryl helped remove the chills and shivering. But next, Keith started getting severe pain in the back. Again, I contacted the oncologist nurse and was advised to administer pain meds. Thankfully, that helped calm the back pain.

It was now October 10, 2019, at the City of Hope again for a new CT scan for Keith. The scan results showed no new growths, and all previous tumors looked stable. We noted on the blood tests the CEA at the City of Hope was seven. It had been thirteen last time. We had hoped this indicated the new therapy regimen worked.

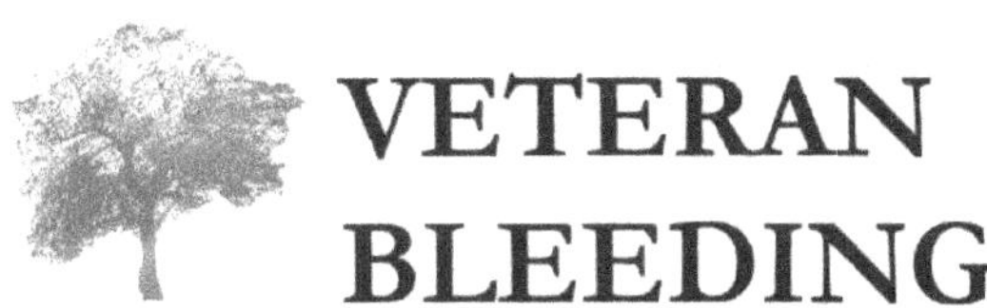 VETERAN BLEEDING

I PRAYED! Once again, I begged! I pleaded to God, and I beseeched the universe! For the life of my beloved husband, who lay in the hospital once again fighting for his life. Again, I pleaded and prayed that Keith was healed entirely and released from his torture. No food for a day and a half. He was bleeding and bleeding. What was the cause? They didn't find the point of the bleed, which significantly worried us. What made Keith's intestines/colon bleed? Why did he bleed and stop and then bleed again? Another day and, hopefully, he wasn't still bleeding. Because if he continued to bleed, they would have opened him up. Keith had suffered enough. The Veteran was bleeding!

Backing up a bit, I must tell more about the bleeding that happened to Keith on, of all days, Veterans' Day in 2019. Keith had an echocardiogram scheduled in Torrance that morning. Afterward, I thought it would be good to go by the mall for a treat and have lunch at one of the food court places. It had been a really long time since we had been to a mall. Keith had used the bathroom before getting lunch. As we sat to eat lunch, I noticed that he was moving slowly and looked a bit pale. I asked if he was doing all right, and he quietly responded that I might have to take him to the ER.

I nearly dropped my food and replied with a big "WHY?" My hunger dissipated quickly when Keith told me he had gone to the bathroom, and it all came out of his backside. His rectum. And, it was bloody and messy. I asked, "Was blood a bright color?" He replied that "it was both dark and bright." Oh geez.

How had he remained calm all that time while we were ordering and getting lunch and sitting down and eating??? I was no longer calm. I was frightened. "Think quick," I told myself. Thankfully, the blood wasn't streaming out of him at that moment, but we had to rush. He was able to walk, so that was good. What should I do? Call for an ambulance or jump in the car and drive him there?

We were only three blocks from the hospital. Wow, I thought this was a plan all along. Perhaps our angels helped us stay around the hospital area because this was going to happen? To once again help save Keith's life. We quickly headed to the car. I asked Keith if we should call for an ambulance. He responded that we could already drive ourselves by the time the ambulance arrived. Keith seemed okay, but I held onto him just in case he fainted from losing the blood. I had no idea how much he had already lost.

We climbed into the thankfully cool car (since I had parked in a covered area) and headed several blocks to the hospital emergency room. It didn't take long to get him into triage to evaluate his needs and assign a room. He had to have a room with a bathroom. Each time Keith felt the urge to use the restroom, the flood of blood came out. I finally saw the toilet and exclaimed that the doctors and nurses also needed to view the scene.

Not to gross you out, but it looked like a miscarriage! Clumps of dark and bright red filled the toilet. Obviously, he was bleeding a lot, but the doctors didn't know where. They finally brought in one of the doctors from Keith's gastroenterology group, and they scheduled a colonoscopy for the following day.

If he were still bleeding, they would clear it out and cauterize the area to stop the bleeding. I wondered why he couldn't do it then and there. I'm guessing they were waiting to see if it stopped. It did! The bleeding finally stopped. Just like a faucet turned off in the middle of running a bath, there was no more bleeding. And no more urge to evacuate from the rectum.

Keith needed a blood transfusion after all that bloodletting. Then a colonoscopy the following day. The gastro doctor met with us afterward and said that he "THOUGHT" the bleeding was from a diverticulum that had burst. He further explained that the colonoscopy (performed at the hospital) didn't find any problems. The doctor suspected a diverticulum had broken off/sloughed off from the inside of the intestine/colon.

But then my thoughts went back to a cancer friend's ordeal with bleeding. This friend had experienced off-and-on bleeding for a while until the problem worsened. He was finally rushed to the hospital, where they tried to operate on him but found there was too much bleeding inside, and they couldn't do anything for him. Could this be happening to Keith?

Yes, our thoughts went instantly to knowing that happened before to others that underwent many years of cancer treatments. Today, I still believe this was the beginning of the end of Keith's cancer saga. Because the week before Keith would leave this world, he again experienced bleeding from the rectum for no apparent reason. But, that last time, there was no carnage, no remains. That time it was bright, fresh blood. And, no transfusions.

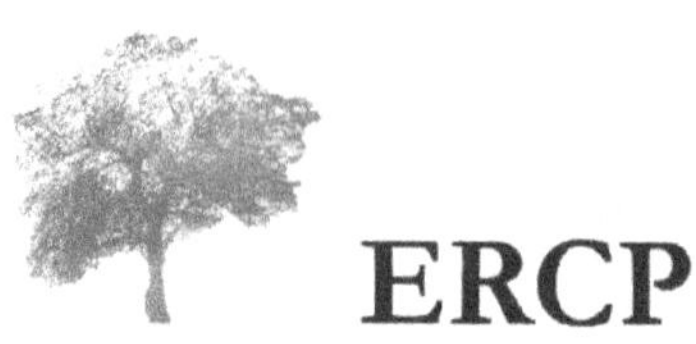

ERCP

I have become significantly concerned. It doesn't appear that Keith feels well at all! He hasn't had much energy to do Tai Chi because it takes an hour of standing. We haven't been dancing either. He stopped writing anything in his cancer journal and he has been concentrating on cars on the computer. This keeps his mind away from thinking about the problem at hand. Why does it seem that he is feeling more and more unwell?

We both knew the answer was his liver. We had watched as the liver numbers alarmingly increased. This was causing liver failure and making Keith feel poorly. But we didn't talk much about it except with the doctors. I know we were both always on the positive track of believing help would arrive at any moment. Just as it had for the past almost eleven years. Meanwhile, we lived the best we could. Keith wasn't very hungry most of the time, so, he began to slowly shrink. We held each other tight and stayed together. We made the best of each day.

It was December 12, 2019, and we were at the City of Hope for a CT. The doctor reported that he had been watching an area, in the liver biliary tree, for the past few scans that seemed to be growing—disconcerting news since Keith had to stop all therapies when the bleeding happened in November. Doctors could administer no therapies since they had planned an emergency ERCP four days later to clear the biliary tree in the liver and alleviate liver failure shown on the blood tests.

"What is ERCP? Endoscopic retrograde cholangiopancreatography, or ERCP, is a procedure to diagnose and treat problems in the liver, gallbladder, bile ducts, and pancreas. It combines x-ray and the use of an endoscope—a long, flexible, lighted tube." Keith's gastro-internist also used a CT machine to assist him in the process.

I am sure most people have no clue what ERCP is. We sure didn't! Check out what I found in researching this interesting subject in the Glossary under ERCP.

December 16, 2019, and yes, we were back to City of Hope for a procedure with a gastro-internist for the ERCP. After the procedure, the doctor brought me into a small conference area and drew a picture of the biliary tree area. He indicated that two cancer lesions were completely encasing the area of the biliary tree! He spoke about how he placed a stent, but he was unsure if it would help. He told me that if that stent failed to alleviate the issue and allow the flow through the biliary areas, the next step would be to place a tube directly through the skin into the liver for drainage. The CT during the procedure showed the bile ducts compressed by the cancer lesions.

After we got home that night, I told Keith what the ERCP physician had relayed to me about how the cancer was compressing the biliary tree. We spoke in an investigative kind of way—Playing out the what-ifs. Should we proceed with the recommended tube if the ducts keep being squeezed? I asked Keith to choose because I would back him up one-hundred percent. I couldn't tell at that time whether he had enough or whether he was still in for the fight.

In case you are curious, Keith and I never talked much about the seriousness of the possibility of dying. We both knew that either one of us could die at any moment. That is life—And death! So instead of being all sappy and hanging onto each other crying, for a possible loss, we sought to be happy instead, even in our trying times. If Keith was up-for-it, we would jump in the car for a short ride to the beach. Just being there at the beach, either sitting in the car and gazing at the rolling ocean tides through the car windows or walking alongside the surfer's beach. Either way Keith and I would get some Earthing to help us on the journey.

On December 21, 2019, Keith was approved and administered the chemotherapy pill Xeloda. Both the oncologist and City of Hope doctors had conference calls and thought it prudent to get Keith on some kind of chemotherapy that his system could take. And, with the stent, they saw a lowering on the blood tests for the liver. Keith began that day (the 21st) by taking these tablets, three in the morning and three at night. Keith had taken these pills long ago and was able to do okay, but this time Keith had problems tolerating the effects.

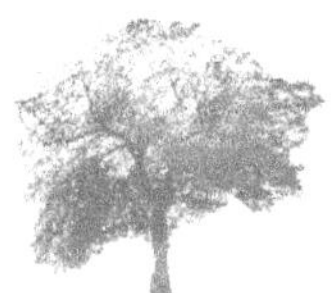

2020

Another year. It was now 2020. It was amazing. It was just 2003, and we were getting married, and then so much had happened since 2003, and then it is 2020. Where had the time gone?

To say the least, Keith and I quite brilliantly captured as much adventuristic times together as one can pile into these years so far. There are copious amounts of ventures that I cannot show in this book. Otherwise, there would be several volumes.

But when experiencing scary times like we were in early in 2020, my mind would wander-off about our many escapades years past. One such adventure was about the time a mouse stowed away in our car after we stayed at our friend's cabin for the weekend.

Picture this: Keith moves a jacket lying on the backseat of our Chevy Equinox. He jumps back quickly when he spies a spry little mouse lying on his back, slumbering away (he was under the jacket). Suddenly the mouse awoke and discovered the frozen Keith staring back at him. A scurrying occurred, and the mouse did not do what Keith had wished—To jump outside the car. Instead, the mouse roared under the seat and buried itself quietly deep inside the vehicle. Keith proceeded to open all the car doors hoping that the critter would find its way out into the wild where it belonged. He finished packing things into the back of the car and making sure anything he placed back there was closed tightly, just in case.

I thought it interesting that day because Keith insisted on driving home. Usually, we took turns, or I drove if he wasn't feeling chipper. After all, we went up to the cabin for some more Earthing and relaxation.

After we arrived home, I found out why he drove. Once we got out of the car, he had me place everything on the front lawn. Nothing would go into the house (and we would keep house doors closed). I quizzed him about why and then he told me about finding the sleeping mouse. The fact was, that he didn't know whether it had left the car or was it still inside the car (or worse in our bags!). I freaked out for sure because I might have been riding in the car with a mouse just running around. We went through everything in the car and on the lawn methodically and did not find a mouse.

But Keith, set up a mouse trap with peanut butter inside the car, just in case. The next morning, the poor mouse was discovered Muerto! The peanut butter did it. We also discovered where the poor mouse had gnawed at the plastic around some windows in his quest to get out. Needless to say, we never went back to the cabin in the mountains. It's okay because the cabin was sold not long afterward.

But back to reality. Again, we were in panic mode. Scary times! One moment we were full of hope. The next, seemingly all hope vanished, but we looked up again, and there was hope again. **Hope never dies**. Not ever!

The City of Hope said things were stable back in September after only one infusion of the antibodies, Herceptin and Perjeta. The oncologist said that Keith needed a chemotherapy drug in conjunction with those antibodies. But delay after delay and uncertainty kept that out of the equation until several days before

Christmas.

That was when Keith's oncologist called him in to begin the chemotherapy. They had delayed the chemotherapy to go along with the antibody meds because Keith's liver showed signs of failing. Plus, there was that scary time when Keith bled through the rectum for a day and night in November.

The chemotherapy began as planned just before Christmas but didn't continue. Keith had his next lab test preparing for the antibody meds scheduled a couple of weeks later. The doctors all put a stop to all infusions as well because the liver failure had worsened!

Shall We Dance

IT IS NOW NEW YEAR'S EVE, December 31, 2019. For almost every year of our married life, Keith and I had attended a New Year's Eve celebration dance. This would be no exception. No matter what, Keith was going to the dance. Things were getting serious. But as we always did, we trucked on. Keith made sure we had reservations for the upcoming dance ball. We met others at the dance, had dinner and champagne and even danced a bit. Keith was still out on the dance floor as my partner doing what he (we) loved. Sure, he didn't move as fast as in the past, but he still danced with style no matter what.

Keith kept busy in-between dances making his way to all his dance friends and chatting it up with them. Later on, I would reflect that that was the last time he saw most everyone there at the dance. There was a time they scheduled a game during the dance. The game involved everyone at each table. Keith sat out the game. He saw that as a time to rest with some of his friends (others sitting it out). With that game, I found that I had to dance with others. This was very strange for me. I rarely danced with anyone else. But in my mind, I thought, "Is this my future?"

That would turn out to be Keith's curtain call at the dances and our last time to dance together. I will cherish forever the memories of that last dance with my prince charming.

The next day, January 2, 2020, the exhilaration of the New Year's Eve celebration dissolved and Keith started experienced more difficulties due to the worsening liver failure. The liver surgeon was contacted and he talked with Keith. The surgeon advised him to go to the ER (emergency at the hospital) if he exhibited fever, diarrhea, or throwing up. Thankfully, Keith didn't have those signs. Nevertheless, Keith began to feel terrible because his liver was failing more. It seemed that, unfortunately, the ERCP performed in December had stopped helping. I tried convincing him to allow me to take him to the ER, but it was the weekend, and Keith told me it was the worst time to go since nothing happens on weekends in hospitals.

As the days transpired, Keith hung on. He would take walks on our driveway to the sidewalk and then back into the house. He wanted to keep up some energy and sometimes a bit of a walk seemed to help him.

January 9, 2020, we found our way back to the specialist at the medical institute, where they took Keith's blood plasma sample in June for a blood biopsy test. The specialist viewed Keith's latest bloodwork and previous lab work results and noted Keith's increasing liver failure. We were hoping for another miracle, but the specialist told us he could do nothing because of the liver failure.

That same day, I drove Keith to his afternoon appointment with his liver surgeon. After reviewing lab work for the past month, the surgeon bluntly told us that if he operated to try to clear the biliary tree, that would undoubtedly end Keith's life, and thus it was not the answer to the problem. He recommended placing a biliary drainage tube directly into the liver. He advised the City of Hope to handle the insertion because the surgeon at the local hospital (doing this type of procedure) opted out because of the prior Y90 treatments on the liver.

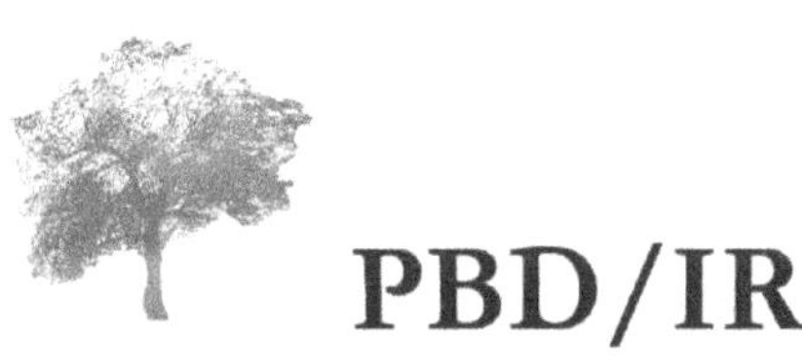

PBD/IR

HOPE was still there for Keith! The City of Hope scheduled a life-saving surgical procedure for Keith on January 14, 2020. City of Hope doctors performed a PBD/IR Cholangiogram Transhepatic. Percutaneous biliary drainage (PBD). Interventional radiology.

Doctors used this procedure to relieve blocks in the bile ducts in the liver. There was a puncture through the body wall and liver for accessing the biliary tree. A catheter was inserted via the biliary tree duct, bypassing the compressed area. The catheter allowed the bile to flow out of the liver, through the skin, and into a bag attached to Keith's leg. The bag had to be drained and measured.

Keith had the PBD surgery to insert the biliary tube. The doctor placed a bag on the outside, and the line emptied into the bag. So that the bag didn't just hang there and pull on the stitches that held the tube on Keith's abdomen, stretchy straps were attached and placed around one leg to hold the bag in place. There was a cup that nurses gave us that had measurement lines, and each time the bag was emptied, I had to measure and note the color of the fluid. Emptying the cup several times daily, went on for nearly two months. And, the entire time, Keith was very much in pain from that bag. As you can imagine, the stitches (holding the tubing) were nudged every which way with the body's movement, especially while trying to sleep.

A nurse would be assigned to come to our home and help flush the tube every day. I was hoping she would also drain the bag, but as it turned out, draining the bag was needed more often than the nurse was here. So yes, I helped Keith with emptying the bag. Each time Keith's bile bag filled up, we rushed to the bathroom. I would uncover the end of the tube and point the tube best we could into the measuring cup. Sometimes the line had a mind of its own and would spurt on the floor or elsewhere. Cleaning brown or green bile (it would change colors by day, which frightened the hell out of us) was not a thrill for either of us. But then it could have been worse.

Note that the average adult excretes between 400-800 cc's daily of bile. After Keith received the bag coming from his liver, on the first full day that I measured each drain, it measured 750cc for that day. The next day it rose to 1225. For the next month, the count slowed until the flow pretty much dwindled to a mere 200cc for the entire day on the last day he would have the tube, March 9, 2020. It had started out good, but something again slowed down the flow to a trickle and made Keith's liver failure worse each day.

Even after Keith had the tube put in, he was back at the City of Hope so that their surgeons could try to re-route some biliary ducts internally to help improve the flow!

We were still hopeful. We remained positive. The tube was supposed to help the liver eliminate the toxins building up inside and causing the liver failure. And, of course, the liver failure made Keith feel poorly. The doctor inserted the tube on the 21st of January. Keith had labs done on the 24th of January, and the bilirubin test had improved from 3.0 to 2.4. At that time, the bilirubin test (one of the liver functions tests) was good enough to start Keith again on Xeloda (the pill chemotherapy).

Keith would start slow and work up to taking three pills in the morning and, twelve hours later, take another three pills. On the following Monday, he was due for another infusion of the antibody meds, Perjeta and Herceptin. The Xeloda made Keith feel undoubtedly more ill, and he fought that feeling like crazy doing all that had helped him get through nearly eleven years of experiencing different types of chemotherapy and other treatments.

By the way, we found out that Genentech agreed to pay for the antibody drugs, Perjeta and Herceptin! Medicare and supplemental denied approval because the drugs were targeted cancer therapy for breast cancer and not for colon cancer! Keith's oncologist office had special people that went way beyond the call of duty and found ways to get the pharmaceutical companies to help. The office staff never gave up.

January 27, 2020, Keith was at his oncologist's office for Herceptin and Perjeta infusions. The week after these infusions, his liver failure numbers raised. At that time, Keith had weekly blood testing. The doctors knew the infusions could influence liver failure. It was a crazy deal trying to kill the cancer without making the liver failure worse and killing the patient!

It was February 11, 2020, and Keith was not doing well at all. I urged him to try to walk since I saw fluids beginning to build up on his legs. But he had zero energy, and he was eating very little. He told me that he never felt hungry. He enjoyed fruit cups of chopped peaches and pears. He did not want to drink the Boost nutritional supplement I got him.

On February 18, 2020, Keith experienced significant heartburn after receiving Xeloda. He couldn't take anything like Pantoprazole because it would counteract the effectiveness of Xeloda. He was allowed to take TUMS. We then found out that the stomach needed to be acidic for Xeloda to work! Oh, joy!

Keith was also suffering from a nasty rash on the shins of both of his legs. We found out that it was a side effect of Xeloda. Interesting that Keith did not suffer the rash when he took the chemotherapy drug long ago!

Keith's edema and fluid retention increased more in his legs and moved to the other parts of his body. The oncologist prescribed Lasik along with potassium. And the chemotherapy pills (Xeloda) and the antibody infusions stopped since liver failure increased again.

It was March 7, 2020, and Keith was still able to move about but very slowly. He had shrunken in size, and his face was sullen, and he had no smile. He had an echocardiogram in the morning, and we attended church in the evening. It would turn out to be his last time attending church. The short walk from the sidewalk into the church and to the pews and back seemed to really wear him out that night.

It was evident with the measuring results of the trickle of bile coming from the tubing from Keith's liver that things inside the liver were getting dire. It was not working at all. Then the weekly blood draws revealed that the bilirubin had alarmingly increased. It really did not make any sense to keep putting Keith through the hell with the tube piercing his side if it was not working. I asked Keith if it was time to remove the tube since it was doing nothing but cause him great pain. He agreed, so, I contacted the City of Hope doctors, and they agreed and scheduled an appointment three days later, March 10, 2020, where they planned to check things out to see what could be done and remove the painful tubing if that was not helping.

March 10, 2020, we were at the City of Hope to see what they could do for Keith's liver failure problem. Lab work revealed that liver failure had increased a lot since last week's labs. The doctors tried to work in the biliary tree area to open the ducts that were being compressed and place stents. Keith was in such misery about everything, including the tube, the doctors decided to remove the tube with the bag. Keith was also given plasma because of his low blood counts. In all his years of so many chemotherapy infusions, he had never had to stop chemotherapy due to low blood counts.

March 13, 2020, a Friday, and I contacted Keith's oncologist to advise him of Keith's greatly deteriorating situation. His body was retaining more fluids even while on Lasik medication. Keith's oncologist recommended taking Keith to the ER (emergency at the hospital) to get Keith checked out. However, Keith refused to go. Keith told me it was Friday night, and he knew nothing happened on weekends. He wanted to wait until Monday.

SERIOUS TIME
PLUS COVID-19 VIRUS
ATTACKS THE WORLD

It was Sunday the 15th of March, 2020, and Keith was not doing well. Fluid retention in his legs and abdomen became an ever-increasing problem in spite of the prescribed diuretics. Before this week Keith tried his best to walk, to hopefully move the fluid out of the body. He walked outside and in front of the house but never went very far. But then, Keith didn't have much energy anymore. His energy had been zapped for a while, especially when he had the tube in his side. But Keith was courageous, as he had been all along. Keith kept up the walking and he moved about until he couldn't. The weekend of the 15th, Keith could barely walk around the house, much less outside.

That Sunday, he seemed to get worse with every hour, and I kept my urging up (that we go to ER) until late Sunday evening (eleven thirty p.m.) when he told me he was cold. I placed another blanket on him and snuggled with him to warm him up. I found Keith was shivering. I had taken his temperature for the past few days as he worsened. I took it then and found it had greatly elevated, yet Keith appeared chilled to the bone, and his teeth were chattering.

I knew from everything I researched and knew that this was not a good sign because it meant he had an infection. Thankfully, he was still in his clothes, so I loaded him into the car as I ignored the continued pleas that he didn't want to go. I drove him to the emergency room at the hospital. I didn't call 911 because he would've told them no, and they would've obeyed. I was hopeful that the hospital could take care of the infection and reduce the fluids he was retaining at an alarming rate.

I was met at the door of the hospital ER and advised that I would only be allowed in the triage area with Keith to give vital information, and then Keith would go to an ER room, and I wouldn't be allowed back there with him in the room. Gosh, I had never let Keith go to ER and be alone. I know how often a person alone in the ER is forgotten. I was fearful for him. But I could do nothing about it. He had to go it alone.

So, I complied, giving the medical staff all the information, I could think of, to help them help him. The team placed Keith in a wheelchair, and I kissed him goodbye and told him, "I Love you," and he said it back to me. I used their restroom and started to look in the waiting room for a seat. I did note that only three people were in the waiting room, so I thought midnight must be a good time. Yes, it was just after midnight on the 16th. But since the COVID protections were in order, I could not wait in the waiting room either.

The guard advised me that I had to go back to my car to wait to see if they would be keeping him. Yikes! I hadn't brought any of Keith's items (phone, charger), just his medical cards to admit him. He wasn't doing too good with his thoughts and he seemed spacey. Probably from the infection his body was fighting.

So, I went back to my car. Thankfully I had driven Keith's car with the soft leather comfortable seats. Lucky for me these seats had warmers on the bottoms and backs, so anytime I got a bit chilled, I just turned on the car for a bit of a warm-up. I soon discovered that the cars next to me also had people inside waiting!

Thankfully, I brought my sweatshirt and down jacket. So I kept comfy (as one can be semi-lying in a car). Hours ticked by, and I didn't sleep. I had my eyes closed, but I kept checking the phone for any messages from the hospital. Nothing. Finally, I had to use the restroom again. Hence, I entered and asked to use the bathroom and also get an update on my husband.

When I came out of the bathroom, a doctor met me and told me that Keith indeed had an infection. They kept him, admitted him to the hospital, and gave him intravenous antibiotics. So, I left to go home. It was after three in the morning. Glad he was being taken care of, but so very sad I couldn't see him and tell him I was going home and that I loved him—Nothing! Nothing and no one had separated us like that before without the chance to exclaim our love for the other.

Early the following day, after barely getting any sleep, I contacted the hospital and found out that Keith also had a blood clot in one leg. We were afraid of blood clots because he had not been able to move about much in the past few days. The nurses had begun a daily injection of blood thinners to break up (safely, hopefully) the clot.

Ultimately, they drained the area around his lungs of fluids but not his belly, scrotum, or legs. His scrotum was the worst. I could not be with him and had to wait at home. So, I was unaware of the scrotum until I got him home. I had no idea everything on his body had expanded significantly.

Wednesday afternoon of March 18, 2020, I received a phone call from the nurse who said she was getting Keith ready to be discharged. The hospital had their first case of the dreaded COVID-19 downstairs, and they wanted to get him and others that could leave the hospital out quickly.

I had heard the converging news about the COVID-19 virus and how more and more people were catching it and landing in hospitals in horrible conditions and even dying. It was scary times, but I had to focus on Keith and not dwell on this new enemy.

I was so thankful that the hospital called me and allowed me to pick up Keith before he was killed by the awful virus or just died there in the hospital without family by his side.

That evening I met my husband and his nurse at the curb. Keith could barely make it into the car. He looked worse than when I brought him to the hospital. His body seemed larger all over.

At home, it was a challenge helping Keith around the house. Keith's huge stump legs appeared painful. His scrotum ballooned bigger than a softball and, he had to hold it up with his hands to help in his tremendous agony. But he refused pain medication.

That night was hard for both of us. Helping Keith walk around the house to get to the bathroom and bed was time- and body-consuming. He could move to pull his pants down, and he had to sit to go to the toilet and hold things down into the toilet. Thankfully, we had gloves on hand. I felt so badly that Keith had to endure so much. Again!

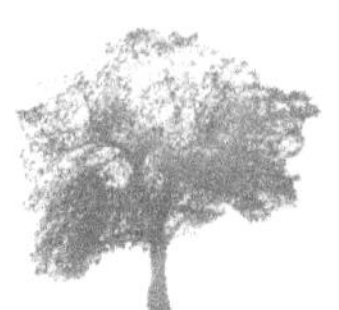

HOSPICE TIME

All I described before was our life until the following night when the hospice representative showed up to set up Keith for hospice care. Keith and his oncologist had settled on hospice while Keith was still in the hospital. Why? Because there was nothing more that could be done for Keith.

Keith was reserved and resigned about his feeling of going into hospice. We both were. We were greatly deflated by the knowledge that this was it. But the reality was there in front of us. Keith's body was tired of the fight. That was very clearly evident with the body's failures. I was numb by then. I think Keith was also. There was no crying or hanging onto each other. I sat with him and we hugged but there were no words or crying. Since we had been through this hospice thing before with others we knew what to expect.

The next day a large delivery truck arrived outside our home. The workers brought in items ordered by hospice; gloves, pull-ups, diapers, adult-sized body wash towels, bed pads, bedside potty, and a bedside patient tray like those in hospitals.

Thankfully, the order included a walker for Keith; the kind that is not so wide (since we don't have wide doorways) and with brakes and a place to sit if needed. It was getting complicated for Keith to get around, so the walker helped a lot. Included with the equipment was a continuous oxygen supply machine on wheels (thankfully) with a long nasal tube so that the device could sit outside the bedroom and the bedroom door shut.

Yes, there was plenty of room under the door for the nasal tube to move freely. Otherwise, it was a noisy machine, and no one would sleep if it were in the bedroom. The delivery men also brought in several backup oxygen tanks as well. It looked like a hospital ward in the house and bedroom.

March 20, 2020: The hospice nurse arrived not long after the big truck to assess Keith. She took blood pressure readings, and surprisingly it was like usual and not too low or too high. She took down all the info for the medication (which the hospice representative had already set up) and asked if Keith wanted to go on morphine.

But Keith quickly told her emphatically that he didn't want to start the morphine because he knew it would put him out, and he wasn't ready to leave reality yet. I didn't push it, but now I wish I had because his condition deteriorated quickly after that. Keith was in great agony. So, to start off, with Keith's approval, hospice began Keith on the lowest dose of Fentanyl for his pain and misery.

They advised Keith that it would help relieve his pain but not put him to sleep. They asked him to let them know if pain increased, and they would get approval for an increase on the Fentanyl. Then the hospice nurse left, and I was there nearly exhausted myself. I don't think people know unless they have done it that taking care of someone nearing the end is an extreme amount of work physically as well as a mental workout.

Feeling overwhelmed, I kept talking with the hospice manager, and finally, we received round-the-clock nursing care for Keith!

Thank God! His condition continually worsened. I became so worn out that I was beginning to wonder if I would go down with him! I also wondered how home care people do this job all the time. It was extremely tough to help Keith. Before all of the equipment, I would walk next to him, holding him and hoping he didn't fall. I knew it wouldn't be likely that I would be able to lift him back up if he did. And helping him in the bathroom was the hardest.

Now, once Keith used the toilet and could stand up, I pulled his pants up (we are talking light sleeper pants). Then, we needed to get him somewhere. At that time, he still wanted to sit on the couch and watch TV. So, I would help him walk back to the living room. The living room was a distance away from the bathroom. Thankfully, he didn't have a weak bladder. Once Keith was ready for bed, that was another ordeal.

We have an adjustable bed, and I would lower it as low as possible. Usually, it was sufficient for Keith to get in and out because it was not high. However, it just became not low enough because Keith was so swollen, he had a hard time just being able to sit on the bed and getting himself scooched back to sit back far enough to turn his back toward the headboard and get his legs on the bed.

Thinking about this, I do this automatically, getting into bed. It shouldn't be so hard. But for Keith, it was. He would get his bottom far back on the bed and start to scoot his backside, and move in the direction of laying his head on the pillow. At the same time, I had to lift one leg and then the other leg and lay each on the bed without squishing his colossal scrotum.

Once there, I elevated the top part of the bed a bit so that he wouldn't lie flat. And, if he wanted, I also boosted the legs a bit. Thankfully, the bed was comfortable. But even so, much of the time from here onward, his misery began to increase. I asked the nurse for more pain meds.

The nurse doubled the Fentanyl. With that addition to Keith's meds, he finally slept. But, later on, I noticed that Keith seemed to become more anxious. Who wouldn't be! So, I asked the nurse for a script of anti-anxiety meds to help. It was impressive that the pharmacy always delivered the prescriptions within a few hours of ordering. It was a unique pharmacy catering to fast and special meds for hospice care.

It was then March 24, 2020, and the round-the-clock nursing care had been a Godsend! I worked with the nurses for everything Keith needed. I was still getting exhausted but not as much as before all the excellent nursing help started. Both nurses (we got one every twelve hours) were obviously dedicated women. I offered them the lounge section of our couch and blankets for sleep at night in between when Keith needed the nursing care.

By the 24th, Keith was no longer getting out of bed and had diapers that needed changing periodically. The nurse in charge, without hesitation, took care of business. I assisted but thanked God again for the help.

The next day, Keith was in bed, and thankfully with the adjustable bed, we could elevate and raise the top enough so that he could eat and drink. He hadn't been eating or drinking much; fruit, yogurt, juice, or water but not much in the past few days. I placed the iPad in front of him to watch TV programs to keep his mind occupied. But he dozed off a lot.

He closed his eyes here and there, and sometimes sleep relieved him of his misery. In the afternoon, I gathered our rosary beads and placed them in Keith's hands, and turned on the marvelous rosary videos they have online—the ones with all five decades of the rosary complete with songs and prayers in between each decade. I recited along with the videos and sang the songs for Keith. Keith always told me he enjoyed hearing me sing. Keith seemed more peaceful listening to the rosary.

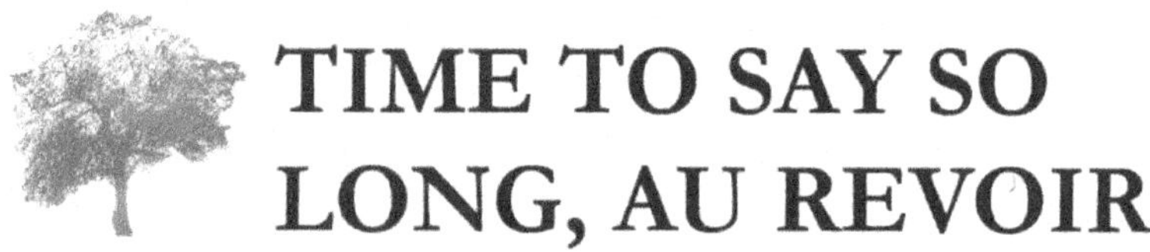# TIME TO SAY SO LONG, AU REVOIR

I felt it. I knew it was time to say, "OKAY, to let go," to Keith.

On that evening of the 25th of March, 2020, Keith seemed to be a lot more anxious, so I requested additional anxiety meds for him. Of course, the nurse on duty received authorization and instruction from the physician in charge of the hospice nurses. Keith could barely move in bed and had to lie on his back the whole time. He hated to sleep on his back, and he usually only slept on his side.

But now, in his predicament, he couldn't even get there (to his side). Keith's body was enormously swollen. Exhausted late that night, I crawled into bed with Keith and lay next to him, holding his swollen hand. Next to him is where I had always slept. Next to him for the past almost seventeen years.

I witnessed and felt his misery. I snuggled up to his side and whispered softly in his ear, "I love you very much, Keith. And, Honey, it is okay to go when you need to go. It is okay to let go and leave." It was extremely tough for me to say those needed words to him without choking and breaking down. I had to hold my tears to get the words said. I needed to let him know it was okay and not to be anxious about staying there with me when he needed to follow the course to his next journey—the time for fighting was no more.

I followed what I had just told him about it being OKAY to go with another saying we used by saying "Now and Forever." Yes, I repeated, "Now and Forever," we would tell each other and write these three words in our greeting cards to each other. We would love each other Now and Forever. No matter here or in Heaven. Now and Forever. I don't know if he could understand me. After I told him it was okay to leave when he needed to, he seemed to respond, but his words sounded like gibberish, and he was tough to understand. I was worried that the drugs affected his brain and did not help his pain. I had already requested morphine the next day.

Afterward, I quietly lay there, listening to him breathing with the oxygen tube in his nose. I lay there and silently cried from witnessing him in so much misery. But I had to stifle my cries lest I upset and make him more anxious.

The tears simply streamed down the sides of my face, dribbling on my neck and dropping onto my nightclothes. I didn't want to move because my hand was still holding Keith's hand, so I lay there with tears moistening my face and neck for a long time. Little did I know that would be the last time I'd be lying next to Keith and holding his hand.

Just as he would seem to relax and sleep, Keith would suddenly start flailing his arms in the air above him. It seemed like the anxiety meds were not doing enough. Keith kept moving his arms up and down from the bed and repeatedly exclaimed, "I AM SO MISERABLE—I JUST WANT TO DIE!" He clearly spoke at those moments. I briefly climbed out of bed to ask the nurse for more medication. She told me she would call for authorization. I got back into bed next to Keith and again held his hand and tried to console him.

Surprisingly, after the flailing, Keith became more restless and clearly told me that he needed to move his body. He hated to be on his back. I offered him my hand and arm to help him readjust where he lay, figuring he just wanted to move just a bit.

But suddenly, he moved a lot more than I anticipated and hurried toward me, trying to get more on his side to face me. At the same time, I wondered if the pain meds were enough in case he squished his swollen body part between his legs? I'm not sure how he did it, but he got almost on his side, and suddenly he let go of my hand, and his heavy arm dropped over my upper body. At that moment, he lay very still, perhaps in fear of what had just happened. I talked to him and asked him if that position was okay. There was no answer. I moved his heavy outstretched arm and spoke again to him louder, calling out his name. No response.

At the same time, as I noticed no response from Keith, the nurse came into the room to give him the authorized meds. I told her what had just happened, and she quickly lowered the head of the bed and helped me lay Keith back on his back to have his vitals checked. She tried to apply the blood pressure cuff on his right arm, but his blood pressure was too low to register.

Did he just pass out? And, he would come to any moment? Then, the nurse startled me by announcing that it was close. Gulp! I realized she meant that he was close to Death. I needed to stay calm and quiet to help the nurse. But, in my mind, I was screaming, "NO, NO, NO." The nurse laid her hand on his chest to feel his heart.

I got up next to him on my knees (still on the bed) and grabbed his wrist to feel for a pulse. I was glad I felt a pulse! But the pulse was not strong and, it grew fainter and fainter, and then it stopped altogether!

I was so shocked by the revelation that his life had ended. But calm at the same time. He seemed to be at peace and not in pain. I couldn't believe it. I just felt his pulse, and then it was gone! I stayed there on my knees on the bed. The nurse also stayed where she was with her hand on his chest. We had to make sure. She wrote down the time: 2:26 a.m. She asked me if I wanted her to handle the call to the mortuary, and I nodded my head yes. I was still in disbelief afterwards and could not find my voice.

I managed to climb out of bed and stood next to Keith. Looking at his serene repose, I saw that he appeared incredibly at peace. I didn't want to do anything, but I leaned down and kissed him on his still, thin, wispy, warm lips. The kiss would be the last kiss here on earth. While bent over to kiss my love, I choked out the words that I loved him as I placed my hand and fingers embracing his warm left hand. I saw his hand, and it reminded me that I had removed his wedding ring before he was admitted to the hospital, and it was a good thing since he was swollen even on his hands.

As I stood looking over my deceased husband, my swallowing entailed deep gulps along with quivering of my lips as I guess I was on the verge of bawling. Traumatized, I stood there still, watching over my dear Keith. I became frozen in shock. My tears finally came after a time. I took a step back to stare at him more. The bed covers still covered his body to his waist. His arms stretched out on both sides of his calm, unmoving body, with his hands lying neatly next to his legs. His face showed no stress, showed no pain. He appeared to be just sleeping, albeit without the chest moving from breathing. Amazingly, his swollen body looked less, as though death had dissolved it all.

I had so many mixed emotions. I was both very sorrowful and happy for Keith at the same time. Because he appeared to be so much at peacetime and out of pain. Keith was at PEACE. Finally! No more torture to try to live another day. And best of all, ultimately, no more painful surgeries and procedures, chemotherapies!

Mentioned in Atul Gawande's book, *Being Mortal*, Plato's *Laches* described Courage as "wise endurance of the soul." When faced with death at the end, Keith had the courage to face the reality of his mortality.

The nurse returned a few minutes later, stopped to hug me, and told me that the mortuary would be there in about forty-five minutes. I felt a new bit of urgency. I realized I didn't have much time with Keith before he was gone from us forever! I quickly opened my great-nephew's bedroom door and woke him to ask him if he would like to say goodbye to his uncle Keith because he had passed away.

My great-nephew jumped out of bed and nearly ran into the bedroom to Keith's side. He turned to me with deep sadness on his face, and we hugged and cried together. James didn't stay too long, and instead, he turned around to say goodbye to Keith, stood there a bit, then went back to his room. He told me later that he buried his head in his pillow and cried for some time afterward. Keith was like a dad to him, so it was important that he say goodbye.

The van from the mortuary arrived about forty minutes after being called. I was surprised to find two big, sturdy men dressed in suits and ties. I was impressed. After all, it was the middle of the night, very early morning. They brought in a gurney as they chatted about how they would be able to transverse around the house and get the gurney in and out. I found they could maneuver the mortuary stretcher into and out of all angles throughout the house. Imagine the stretcher as a robot able to bend everything. Yes, that's how it was. I thought to myself that Keith would've also been amazed at watching the special gurney in action.

Maybe Keith was watching. As some say, about people who have passed on, the spiritual body may hover around a while in the home while getting bearings after passing away and before proceeding elsewhere. I was both amazed and bewildered, along with being so very distraught as I watched the mortuary men enter the bedroom where my very still, pale, dead husband lay quietly on our adjustable bed. I could see them swaddling the white sheets (they had brought with them) around Keith's body and then tying the sheets and then they shut the door.

I guess they didn't want us to watch them place him in the dull black plastic/vinyl-looking bag. The door opened, and the big strapping men began moving the gurney down the long hallway. They had the black bag strapped firmly, so the black bag stayed when they moved any part of the gurney. Once everything was straight, they stopped at the door and asked if Keith was in the armed forces.

I told them, "Yes, the Air Force." They told us they honored all service members, pulled out a regular-sized, neatly folded flag, and draped it over the black bag where my husband lay. The mortuary workers wheeled him to the waiting van and loaded him inside for the ride.

I envisioned them taking him to one of those cold steel areas where they would pull out the long steel drawer, placing his black bag and him inside the drawer. Or perhaps they removed the black bag before putting him in the drawer. I remember wondering that. I was hoping he wouldn't be too cold.

Then the van and the men were gone. Keith was gone! The suffering spent—end of an era. My Superman, our Superman, was gone.

"Your form will simply pass along, but who you really are will never die." (unknown author)

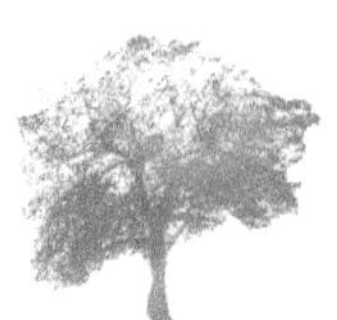# AFTER THE END

For many years (while Keith was fighting cancer), I always outwardly put up the positive front. But, in the back of my mind, I had a feeling that I would someday have to deal with another funeral. Usually, late at night, when I lay there again thinking way too much about my lists of lists, I would contemplate and plan in my mind's eye my great husband's magnificent funeral—Keith's funeral. This remarkable man of mine deserved to be honored, and of course, I wanted him to go out with as much fanfare and style, with my pageantry ways, as we had done for our wedding.

I had envisioned our music director friend playing beautiful music at our local church. I also imagined Keith's flag-draped casket rolling down the aisle for the longest ride to the altar, as it had with Rudy's funeral. This scenario changed when we decided on cremation.

Since the decision to do cremation, I remained somewhat confused on how to plan since I had only attended two memorials where the cremation remains were in a box/container on a table at the front of the church.

I would play it back and forth in my mind—this scenario for the funeral of our beloved Superman. In the "funeral" movie, of my mind, I would try to maintain, try not to cry, try to sing along with the great music but alas, I would always fall apart and succumb to the rolling tears.

I would end my planning thoughts with deep swallows each night as I tried to contain myself. Otherwise, I might wake Keith. I would lay there with tears streaming down the sides of my cheeks until I went to sleep. You see, I was always holding my husband's hand with my right hand. We would fall asleep like that. I could not let go to wipe the tears away from my face.

But for some reason, the last few months of Keith's life, my planning had more or less stopped. I don't remember why it stopped. Perhaps because of the huge transition of the uncertainty of what was happening with Keith's health.

Instead, every night I would spend my non-sleeping time thinking about how the doctors were planning and how treatment didn't seem to be working. Plus, worrying that too much time had elapsed and cancer must have been growing more. Yes, I would find later on that my worries would be the truth that would become Keith's demise.

So much for plans. They all went down the drain with the COVID-19 pandemic. There would be no beautiful music, nor would there be a funeral. And, I was only allowed to make mortuary and cemetery plans once Keith passed away.

Yes, I know you all will say why didn't we already have funeral plans? We thought about it several times over the course of many years. But Keith had been lucky, with so many miracles and Hail Marys, so we thought he had a lot more time. Part of us also thought that if we made funeral plans ahead, that would be giving in. We were so wrong. We had run out of time.

When Keith came home from the hospital for the last time, I finally saw the writing on the wall. He wasn't going to make it much longer. I called right away and made appointments with two mortuaries. Thankfully, I attended the first appointment and concluded that they wanted so much money, it was almost ridiculous.

I talked it over with Keith and planned to make the next appointment for the other facility the following morning. However, that appointment did not happen. The mortuary called that night and advised that no more arrangements were allowed—only once my husband passed away. I couldn't make any plans at all ahead of time. I had only a slight idea after talking with the second company on the phone about their pricing.

I had to decide to go with them sight unseen, or what? What a pickle we had gotten ourselves into while not planning ahead for this. I was thankful that although we did not speak of death, Keith and I just knew what would happen, and we talked more in-depth about a place for Keith. He gave me his idea of where and told me to make the final decisions.

So, in the middle of the night, early at two thirty a.m. on that Thursday in late March, 2020, with my unimaginable grief, I had to make a quick decision when asked where my husband's body would go, which mortuary. Thankfully, I chose the other morgue that I had not viewed. Would I regret this decision? Thankfully not.

Keith was at peace. Finally, no more torture to try to live another day. Finally, no more pain and procedures, no more chemotherapy or surgeries to cut away his body trying to make things right. Keith was Free!

"I'm Free

Don't grieve for me, for now, I'm free; I took His hand when I heard Him call; I turned my back and left it all." (Robert Burcham)

The quote above I picked for Keith's memorial handouts. Anyone trying to plan a funeral when they have just lost their spouse understands that you will most likely be in a brain fog of epic proportions. It is best to bring a support person to help you finalize everything. It is unbelievably the most challenging thing to do—plan a funeral. Most especially after I found that there would not be even a funeral anywhere as the government had just shuttered everything, including churches.

There would not be an on-site burial either, but the cemetery personnel told me that I could have a small gathering of ten people. I muttered to myself, "OK, I can deal with that."

Honestly, I could not fathom there would be no funeral at all to honor my beloved Superman, and with no on-site burial service, where would these ten people go, and what would we do to honor Keith?

A few days later, the cemetery people phoned me and told me that only burial prayers would be allowed and only in the parking lot, and only two people would be allowed. I broke down in tears on the phone when they told me that.

My Keith would not be receiving anything at all. My nephew overheard me crying and came over and placed his arm around me, trying to comfort me.

The mortuary kept changing plans almost by the hour. One moment they called to tell me there would be an honor guard with a trumpet and folding of the flag, but then that got nixed altogether the night before the burial.

During an additional call the night before the burial, the cemetery told me that I could have five people in the parking lot, and everyone would need to stay in their cars. I called my brothers to see if they wanted to join me and my nephew.

But, in one of their cars, since only two per car was allowed. I then got the priest to set up between us, close enough to hear the priest. Thank God for the brave priest.

On the day of the burial, I had to drive myself and my nephew in our car. Driving myself to my husband's burial was not something I relished. Our vehicles lined up on either side of a small altar set up in the parking lot facing the building. The weatherman had predicted rain, but instead, it was a lovely sunny morning with beautiful clouds above, sort of lighting the parking lot where we waited. When the priest walked and stood in front of the altar (that was between our cars), we opened our side windows so that we could hear the priest speak. Thankfully, it was not too chilly.

Meanwhile, a finely dressed man from the cemetery brought the box with Keith's remains in a colorful, soft-appearing velvet bag toward where the priest stood waiting. The finely dressed man removed the golden metal box and placed it on the stand in front of the priest next to the long-stemmed red roses I had handed to the priest previously.

I remember watching as the man placed the golden box on the prayer stand that held a place for a bible/book/papers and holy water to bless the box. I remember all this, but I was in my death-suffering fog. So, I didn't come to terms that it was Keith's remains inside the box right away. I was also in the mode of having a job to do and driving the car where my nephew sat. That all kept me from falling apart right there in the car.

As we all strained to hear, the Good Father said the prayers and spoke a few minutes and, when all was said and done, he asked that we remain in our cars as he accompanied the cemetery men up to place the box in the assigned place.

I watched as a spiffy-dressed Latino man lifted the shiny copper metal box with the flowers and the beautiful, soft, velour matching bag that came with the cremation container. He carried it ceremoniously into the mausoleum building. That building is open throughout the floors so that it has no walls and no windows. The wind rushes through everywhere. I imagine the marble allows it to stay cool even in hot summers. Hopefully, I will be allowed to visit my husband's resting place and bring him flowers by summer. Since it was so open everywhere in that building, I wondered why we were not allowed to go up there with Keith.

It didn't seem very long before the priest returned and told us he had spoken the appropriate prayers and watched as they placed Keith's box in the assigned area and closed it. The Father reported that he then put the flowers in the tiny flower vase attached to Keith's final resting place. I knew that it would be a very long time before the government removed the restrictions and I could visit Keith. And it would be a very long time before they installed Keith's name plaque. Since the COVID-19 virus squelched so many jobs all over the country, everything stopped or slowed to a crawl.

After the priest completed the burial and departed, we left to go home for breakfast. It would have been nice to go to a restaurant after the burial. But due to the virus restrictions, nothing was open for dining. Food places only allowed food picked up. Instead, I prepared breakfast for my nephew, two brothers, and myself (although I was not hungry), and then we all set about moving James entirely to his new apartment.

Yes, the same day I buried my husband, I moved my nephew out of the house to an apartment. That is another story in itself. But the short and sweet of it was that Keith wanted him moved and living on his own, and the day after Keith passed away, I got a call that the agency helping my nephew had an apartment for him. Yes, I had to handle all of this at the same time. Maybe it helped me cope, or perhaps it stressed me out even more.

"It is done. "At the end of that day, that is what I said. Maybe out loud. I can't remember. "It is done." My great-nephew, was moved and out of the house. My husband was gone. He was no longer suffering. His long fight over. It was unbelievable. We thought for sure this would be just another bump in the road, and someone would save Keith as it had happened before in the past eleven years. I still can't believe he is gone.

"I was enveloped by the stillness, emptiness, and loneliness that are companions to death." (Nancy Guthrie, 2005).

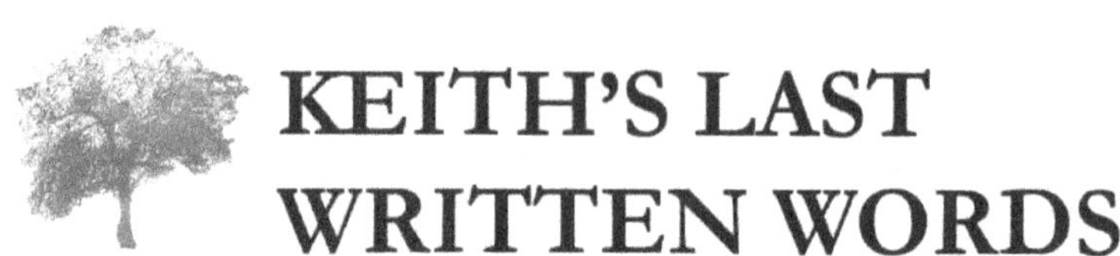

KEITH'S LAST WRITTEN WORDS

Keith wrote this in his journal a few years ago as his last entry. I saved this for his last words.

My hope is that if this story helps anyone out there, then praise the Lord, for he is great. I have been blessed, and I admit that this has been a very hard journey, but I could not have made it without GOD and without my wife.

If any of you think you can fight Cancer on your own, don't even try because you will lose. Cancer is a tough hard battle, and without someone in your corner, you cannot fight this fight alone. The power of prayer (ask everyone you know or meet because the more prayer, the more GOD hears) and a support team is very important for fighting this disease.

Here is what I suggest: Pray all the time. Every day, every evening, pray to God that clearing the cancer and living a long, happy life is God's will. Ask others to pray for you. Be sure to have someone at your side at all times to help you fight the battles with the medical personnel when you are too weak to fight.

Be always proactive in your care so that you don't go through the pains I endured at the hands of people who shouldn't be treating cancer patients. Learn everything you can by asking or researching on the internet.

You will receive information from friends, relatives, and strangers because everyone wants to help you. Remember that everything you read is not always going to be true or helpful. You have to learn to sift through everything you read or hear to know the real truth or to understand what you need to do for yourself to make it through this bumpy life journey.

One thing is certain—tough times never last, but tough people do last. Think as a Super Man and you will become a Super Man and a John Wayne and whoop the Big C's butt! Au Revoir! Adieu!

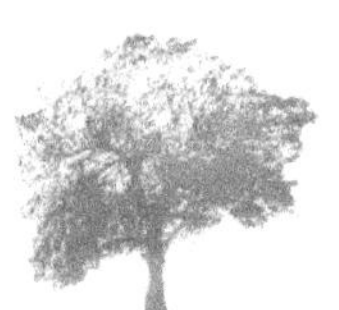

THE REALITY

I was genuinely "crushed with grief." (NLT 1996). Inconsolably brought down to the core, to the lowest point of my being, and feeling as if I too was at death's door. When asked how I was doing after my husband's death, I would tell people, "Fine." But deep within me, my soul felt incredibly crushed, overly consumed, with gut-wrenching and unbelievable deep pain. Along with the gripping soul pain came the uncontrollable outbursts.

First, there was the pressure to contain myself. The pressure would begin to build. Then, I held my breath for fear of bursting at the seams. It would be so intense that it would almost take my breath away. Then the tears would burst forth with a vengeance and seem to flow forever. I thought I would feel better after tears. But then more tears. The uncontrollable sobs, the quivering lips, and quiet moans.

Even though a bit of time had passed (almost two weeks), I did, at any given moment, experience a déjà vu of the intense trauma of Keith's death and re-experienced the incident as if it just happened.

As I woke up that cloudy April mid-morning, I tried to focus and clear my eyes. Part of me wanted to go back to sleep. After all, rest was hard to come by the night before, as it had been most nights since Keith died. However, the realization soon set in, and, in my bereavement, I once again grasped that I buried Keith the day before. Almost two weeks after he transitioned. When the essence of Keith was no more, and only his earthly body remained.

I also realized that day was my birthday, and now I was totally alone. With so much going on, I had forgotten about this birthday. It should've been a big deal turning seventy and all. But now, this birthday was meaningless.

As I mulled over about how I should at least get up and start my day, I thought about how messed up things were with my situation and the entire world. It was COVID-19 virus time. People were dying every day everywhere in the world.

The deadly COVID-19 virus kept everything at a standstill. Suppose I had wanted to celebrate my birthday (which I did not), no celebrations or gatherings were allowed. No one could come over, nowhere to go, and nothing was open. We were all at "stay at home" status—the most unbelievable of times.

Deeply depressing times.

I don't remember being this depressed. Even with Rudy's death (my second husband), I mourned for a year or more **before** his passing away. I was in a fog for a while after he died, but I don't remember this deep depressive mood that I was experiencing with Keith's death. Perhaps because with Rudy's death, I had friends and family surrounding me constantly afterward. They kept me busy, took me places, and spent time with me. And they kept my mind from being too depressed while I was with them.

But not this time. My friends could not come to visit. My only relatives were my two brothers and my nephew. So, my only connection with friends and distant relatives was through texts and social media. AND there were NO hugs—those hugs one needs after going through a death of a husband. That drove the depression deeper and deeper.

I stayed numb and emotionally overcome by profound grief. The reel of life and death played over and over in my mind. And the rush of reality would come to me, again and again—that he was gone. Keith was dead. He was gone!

It was hard to grasp. It was hard to realize that Keith's spirit and soul departed from his body and our earthly environment. I wondered then, and I wondered later if he was floating above his body, close to the ceiling, viewing what was going on below him in the room(s)? Or was he whisked off to the white light, to the outstretched arms of his waiting parents on the other side? Would he contact me, as Rudy had done in the past? I would find out later.

Did I expect this? Not really. We believers just never gave up HOPE. Never! Miracles had happened so much in Keith's life. Many! But that was his time to go to Heaven. He was out of pain. No more misery, thank God. Now more grief began for me. The love of my life, my real soulmate, was gone.

Thinking back on the morning of Keith's passing, I remember after the mortuary van and the hospice car drove off, the house became incredibly quiet. I didn't think I should go back to the bed that Keith had just died in and lie down and sleep. So, I took to the couch and curled up among my easy-down blankie. I hugged it like one would embrace someone, or perhaps I was hugging the spirit of Keith. Finally, the roaring tears overtook me. Waves and waves of overwhelming grief and outright sobbing took me to the depths of my being.

After what seemed like a long time sobbing and finally calming the sobs, I knew sleep would not come. So, I thought I'd reach out to everyone online and let them know about the tragedy. After all, we communicated quickly via email or social media in those times. I certainly was not up to personally calling everyone we knew to tell them. I was an emotional wreck already.

We had our email system set up to send one email to everyone in specific lists (emails) already preset. Therefore, I set out to prepare a statement to "Keith's Prayer Lists." It was most difficult writing a letter to everyone about my husband dying in my arms! While trying to focus through my on-again streaming tears, I managed to type and send the notification email letter and requested prayers for Keith's soul. Thank goodness for the ease of email.

After the letter, I went back to the couch, curled up, tears still streaming, unbelieving what had happened. I kept repeating out loud, "what the hell, what the hell." I still couldn't believe that he was gone. Keith was gone from the bed where we slept side by side, holding hands—gone from the home we shared for the past almost seventeen years. Gone from life. Gone from MY LIFE. "Oh, My God!" I found myself exclaiming over and over.

Needless to say, I still did not sleep after that. After closing my eyes for a brief time, my eyes were jarred open by the sounds of texts and messages from people who had gotten up back east and sent forth sympathy words. Reading those helpful, kind words just got me choked up again.

Weeks later, I would find Keith's little calendar on his desk. Keith had a small personal daily calendar with prayers and sayings for each day. When Keith went to his desk, he would flip the calendar to that day and sometimes read me the small, heartwarming quotes. When I saw the small calendar and what day the page showed, I was flabbergasted! Keith had not been able to move from his bed for the past three days before he died. He also had not been in our office for at least five or six days before he passed. But, yet, his calendar sat already flipped to March 26th! The 26th—the early morning that he died! Did he know? Or did his angels move the calendar to the day of his last breath? I am not making this up—just read what the calendar said for March 26th.

God—sometimes I find the path to YOU rocky and difficult, and I often stumble. I need to remember that each uphill step brings me

Hunt for the good point of your friends. Remember, they have to do the same in your case. MARCH 26

Wow! This prayer of sorts sounded like a prayer Keith would make on his last day of his life. His road home WAS extremely difficult!

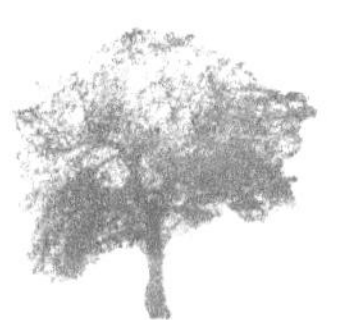

TWO WEEKS SINCE

It had been a few weeks since Keith felt the nudge of the others (to join them on the other side), the urgency of God, to take his leave and go. Was there a white light he followed? Keith must have known something was about to happen. I wondered. Because on Keith's final night, as I lay next to him on his left side, I suddenly felt him trying to wiggle his bottom to move even closer to me.

He was moving quickly and trying his hardest to get on his side with his arm stretched toward me. I now believe he was making his last movement to hug me once more before leaving this plane. He must have felt something and known that he was dying. Keith scooted, moved to his side, and deliberately moved his arm over to my left side.

As soon as Keith's arm reached my whole body, his arm fell heavily across my chest and side with his hand on my left arm as if to embrace me. He was hanging onto me—my last hug! He did not want to leave me! But he had to!

Being enveloped in a thick veil of cognitive fog ever since, back then, as I stood in my bedroom facing our long closet, I opened the long, sliding, mirrored closet doors, revealing empty shelves throughout. The cleared-out shelves stared at me with the same haunting silence that I felt throughout the house and my soul. The shelves were empty because my friends had just taken away a lot of my husband's clothes to a clothes bank on the west side to help the church ministry in the area. My soul was just as empty as those shelves—the Keith connection lost. The human connection to my dear departed husband, Keith.

As I peered at the empty white shelves, I felt the loss once more. Gulp, I took a swallow. My eyes welled up and overflowed down my face. I grabbed my face with my quivering hand over my mouth and cried uncontrollably. Again.

It was unquestionably unbelievable that I was living this loss. It was incredible that it happened at all! Keith was supposed to kick this cancer. He was supposed to survive. After all, we had dubbed him Superman back in 2010, the first time we celebrated when told he had kicked cancer.

Since we never really talked to each other about his (Keith's) impending death, we just understood. We had been through so many deaths together; long ago, his mother, my dad, and then my mom a few years ago. It was as if we were speaking through our minds. We just knew.

We didn't want to talk about it with our mouths because our senses would overwhelm us, and we would each fall apart. We each seemed to feel the need to be strong for the other. But that is the way we did it for the long eleven-year journey. Motor through, keep it going, keep on swimming (as Dory would say in the movie *Finding Nemo*).

I don't know how exactly. But I felt Keith's time here on earth coming to a close, maybe starting in November when he had the mega bleeding incident. But I relaxed and told myself he still had some fight left. Then came the annual New Year's Eve dinner dance.

I noticed Keith running out of energy often. The first of 2020 was when his liver failure was not showing very many signs of improvement. Then I knew in March that the torture far outweighed the results. Keith had suffered long enough. But still, Keith wanted to fight and did not show signs of giving up or letting go.

It must have been his last stay in the hospital the week before he passed when I let everyone know at the hospital (and his doctors) that they would not make Keith suffer any longer. The doctors knew and finally let Keith know (and I know Keith already knew) that there wasn't anything else they could do for him. There would be no more miracles.

But, alas, when Keith's doctors told him time was up, I couldn't be with Keith, at the hospital, because of the COVID-19 virus. He was alone in the hospital when the oncologist met with Keith and his liver doctor. I imagine they both had tears in their eyes as they spoke with Keith and more or less said their goodbyes.

The oncologist called me afterward to relay the conversation. In an emotional voice, he told me that Keith had not been just his patient all those years but a friend and that they had been through so much together in the past eleven years.

At a certain point, I had gotten Keith (via nurses) his cell phone for use in the hospital, so it would be easier for him to contact me. After he met with the doctors, we spoke, and he told me that there wasn't anything else they could do. He seemed resigned, okay, and he had come to terms with it.

I was sorry I wasn't able to be there and hold him. We did Facetime, and the hospitalist doctor came in, and we discussed his condition and how the liver failure was making him fill up with fluids. Of course, I was concerned with his situation and wanted comfort for him, but he refused anything like morphine.

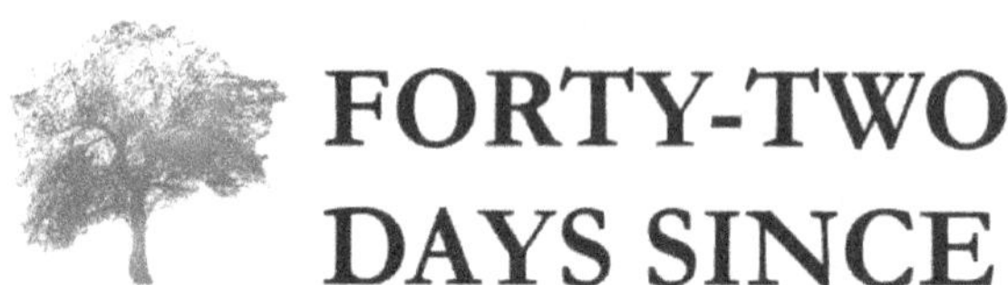# FORTY-TWO DAYS SINCE

It was forty-two days since Keith left this earthly physical world. There was no kidding anyone. It had been damn tough. I guess I just thought things would be different, and there would be a final cure for his cancer, and we could live on together. I was hopelessly disappointed that Keith wouldn't be here to share my life with me.

About three weeks after Keith's death, I started having this obscure, strange ear problem on the left side of my hearing. I was hearing swooshing sounds to the beat of a heartbeat! My own heartbeat? Since I had never experienced this before, I didn't know what to expect, and thus, I became incredibly distraught. Extreme mourning conditions were overwhelming me, and I was beginning to be indeed fearful that it was causing health problems. The sounds in the left ear were all-consuming, mostly at night.

They seemed to grow more and more in loudness. With that, my anxiety rose as well. Sleep was hard to come by. Calming apps helped a bit. Finally, I went to the doctor for advice and saw an ear specialist. That specialist tested everything and pronounced it to be tinnitus. My problem was with the ear and the noise only because I could hear fine. The problem was extremely frustrating.

As an after note, written a year later, I researched like crazy to solve this problem ever since. The noise dissipated a bit but was never totally gone. Perhaps my level of anxiety had decreased, and thus the noise reduced? I also found a medical study whereby they discovered that a person undergoing humungous amounts of stress could suddenly experience effects on the brain that can bring tinnitus to the ear—the results can stay long term or dissipate altogether. I pray for the latter.

While I contemplated my new life, I thought about Keith, of course. And, I wondered if he was there in Heaven talking about all the Bible stuff he knew. He always read the daily readings and history of the saints and the church. Of course, one year, he got a particular Bible and read it every day for an entire year when he finally completed reading it.

I was so proud of him. It reminded me of when I was a young girl, and my Grandpa Mordecai (on my father's side) told me he would pay me with a brand-new one-hundred-dollar bill to read the whole Bible. Of course, I had no idea what a one-hundred-dollar paper bill looked like, but it sounded terrific, so I tried. I tried to read the Bible at a young age (not sure, but guessing between seven to ten years old), keeping my attention and reading the strong Bible text was tricky.

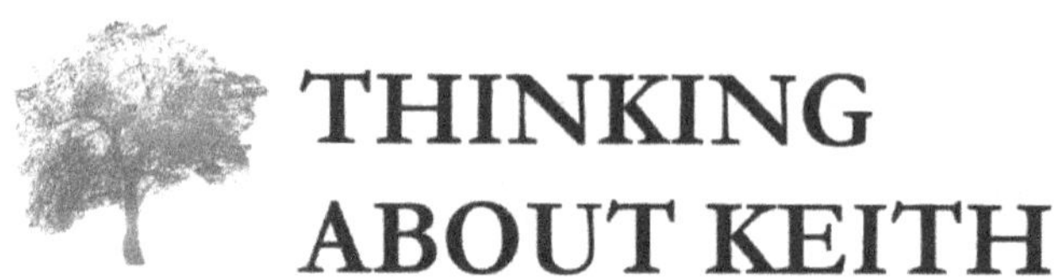

THINKING ABOUT KEITH

B ut, again, I digress as I wanted to talk about Keith.

In thinking about Keith, I wondered why I was not "hearing" from Keith anymore. You will know what I mean once I explain further. You see, Keith had contacted me. Yes, you might think I'm some sort of nut, but it all makes perfect sense. I knew if he could figure it out, he would pull it off, and he did. A year before Keith passed, we talked about this very same thing—about Keith contacting me after he passed away. It was a normal conversation and nothing heavy. I had asked Keith, "How will I know it is you that is contacting me and not my late husband Rudy contacting me?" Keith told me he would figure it out, and hopefully, there would be something else he could do to let me know without a doubt.

Before telling about my experience of Keith contacting me, let me fill you in a bit about my other late husband, Rudy. Before Keith, there was Rudy.

I told you a bit previously about my second husband, Rudy. Rudy passed away in 1992 after suffering from acute congestive heart failure for almost two years. The congestive heart failure situation began a few months after he survived a quadruple bypass plus an aortic valve replacement in 1990. Rudy suffered a lot in his last years, losing so much weight throughout those final years that I had to keep buying him clothes.

He demanded to wear stylish clothes and be best dressed always no matter what. He also insisted on walking around the corner to work even though he was gravely ill. He was getting indeed hateful and downright demanding and mean in his last few months of life. All I wanted to do was love him. It was a challenging time. Then the funeral and the burial at the plot he had purchased long ago.

A day or so later, after the funeral and burial, the happenings with Rudy started occurring.

We lived in a company-owned rented house on the street behind where we both worked. Rudy was the CPA. The company owned the house, and they intended to demolish the property to use it for something else. But once they heard we needed to rent a home, they fixed up the house for us to move in. Renovations included rewiring the house entirely. Everything had been inspected and passed. We had no problems with electricity after we moved in. That is until Rudy died.

Then, we also had a very close-by adjacent bathroom in our bedroom. The bathroom light and fan came on simultaneously and activated with the same switch. The fan made a loud growling noise, so I could hear the fan come on when the light turned on.

I had trouble sleeping after burying Rudy. In fact, it was hard going to sleep and difficult staying asleep. Several nights passed since I buried Rudy and, I think I was probably lightly sleeping when I realized the loud fan sounding in the bathroom. I woke up more as the noise continued. For some reason, I didn't feel alarmed. I knew I hadn't just left it on before going to sleep because I could never sleep with that darn fan sound blaring. I got up and opened the bathroom door and turned off the light\fan switch, and went back to sleep, wondering what had just happened. Even today, I can still recall those strange happenings.

The following nights, the same thing happened. In the middle of the night, I would wake to the fan's brash noise in the bathroom. The light/fan turning on by itself didn't happen every single night but consistently sounded many times for several weeks, and then it stopped and never happened again, there. Meanwhile, at the same time as the bathroom happenings, in the family room where I had left Rudy the day he passed away, there was a lamp on a wooden end table next to the couch where Rudy usually sat.

After Rudy passed, I sat at that end of the sofa, next to that lamp. I guess it was comforting for me to sit where he used to sit. For a while (like every other day for a week), that lamp would turn on all by itself. Usually, when I would leave the room and return, it would be on. And then, after the last time, it also stopped. I never had the light go on by itself again while I lived there. And, once I moved to the next two living quarters over many years' time span, it never happened. But I kept using the lamps. Rudy had just purchased them before we moved. They were brand new and we never had the lamps turn on by themselves before Rudy passed away. The lamps were the very expensive durable touch types that were just coming to the stores.

Now, one would wonder and ask me, "Weren't you at all scared out of your wits with the fan noise going on in the middle of the night? And, the light in the family room turning on by itself (usually during the day)?" And I would tell you that I didn't feel fearful at all. And, I didn't feel any alarm. I cannot explain it entirely, but I felt calm. I also immediately thought that it was Rudy. I instinctively knew that he was angry at me for not cremating him and saving money.

After having difficulty obtaining sleep, I would actually talk to Rudy in the middle of the night because he would invariably wake me. I would admonish him out loud, yelling, "Rudy, why are you waking me with the fan? If it's about not doing the cremation, I'm sorry, but you have the plot at Forest Lawn and would never talk about things, so I had to make my own decision!"

Even today, I believe that was Rudy that kept turning on the lights and the fan.

Years later, it was also Rudy that contacted me the night before my dad was dying. Rudy loved my dad, and they got along almost like brothers. So, when my dad was on his last days at age ninety, dying of a hole in his intestine and lying in a hospital room with morphine coursing through his veins to relieve the intense pain, it was Rudy that signaled me. I'm sure of this. Rudy also contacted me when I married Keith.

Just so you know, after Rudy died, I moved to a rented condo in Torrance. No non-assistant light-on happenings there. After a few years, I next moved to my condo in another city. Nothing happened there either regarding lights going on by themselves. Two places I lived and no "lighting" contact. Yes, I still had and used the same lamps.

But, when I got connected with my new husband, Keith, and moved in with him, that's when it happened again. The lights going on by themselves started just a week or so after we got married. I had moved in my things and yes, the lamps were included and needed in our bedroom. For a couple of weeks or more, the lamp next to my side of the bed turned on in the middle of the night without assistance. I had some explaining to do.

Keith had thought I kept leaving the lights on and said he would not have slept through it, so I think he finally believed my stories about Rudy making the lights go on long ago in my rental house with Rudy. Yes, it was the same lamps. We both had a lamp next to us on either side of the bed. Now, mind you, I had had the lights previously all checked out and made sure they didn't have a short. Electrical technicians said that my lamps were expensive and would last forever, plus the lamps had absolutely no problems.

Being a master of all things electrical, plumbing, and the like, Keith set about to figure out the problem with the lamp. He found no problem with the lamp or the electrical outlet on my side. Yes, the lights on incidence only happened to the lamp next to my side. Then, like the previous lights-on incidents, they stopped. I told Keith that I felt that Rudy told us that he approved of our marriage.

You see, I really believe Rudy had dealings in helping us find each other and getting us together. I was wildly convinced because when I met Keith and saw his lovely home, right away in my mind, I declared that Rudy would have loved Keith's home with all the built-in wood bookcases and showcases. It was an actual calming effect just knowing that my previous deceased husband had possibly helped put us together and was happy about the union.

Still talking about the light phenomena business, I fast-forward many years later. Eighteen years after Rudy's death and seven years after my marriage to Keith, my ailing, frail, ninety-year-old father lay in a hospital, dying of a perforated intestine. The time is 2010, and Keith had been fighting cancer for the past year. So, I had to divide my time between my ailing father and my ailing husband. After an afternoon and evening at the hospital where my father lay, I left late at night when my brother came in to relieve me. I made sure the nurses administered morphine to help my father with his heavy pain. Early the following day, around two thirty a.m., the light came on in the lamp by my bed, and I was awoken by Keith poking at my back, telling me Rudy was calling.

I was so exhausted I just turned the light off and went back to sleep. Around three a.m. the light was back on, and again Keith nudged me awake. Still, I turned the light off, and slumber commenced. Later, about four a.m., the light came on the brightest, and Keith shook me, telling me it must be urgent because the light is on its brightest setting. Finally, I figured out Rudy was trying to get me to the hospital for my dad. So, I rushed to the hospital with my rosary beads.

I arrived at the hospital to find my dad writhing and flailing his arms in what I thought was pain. I notified the nurse and wondered how long it had been since anyone had checked on him. I had left him around eleven p.m. when my brother was there, and he was going to stay awhile, but obviously, we all had to go home to sleep.

The nurses said they had given him morphine, and he wasn't due for another, but they thought he wasn't resting comfortably. Instead, his nerves were reacting, and he wasn't calm. They gave him a calming medication, and he seemed to relax finally.

I spent the next couple of hours with my dear father, moving my fingers up and down the rosary beads with my right hand and the other hand under the blanket, holding my dad's soft, worn hand clasped in mine. I recited the rosary prayers as my tears streamed down my face and dropped on the bedding before me. It seemed to appear to be his end time, and I was very emotional. At one point, I could swear my dad squeezed my hand, giving me a sign that he was comforted with the prayers. My dad died later that morning after my mother arrived. I figure he was waiting for her.

Of course, I said a prayer thanking Rudy for waking me to come to help my dad early that morning. And, now was it Rudy again contacting me after Keith passed? Or was it Keith who had figured out Rudy's ways?

Keith Contact?

SINCE KEITH INVOLVED HIMSELF with spiritual healing during his long eleven-year cancer battle, I had no problem believing he would find a way of contacting me. Of course, I know you probably thought I was making this up. But why would I? There is absolutely no reason. Everything actually happened, as I stated. I had inclinations in the spiritual realm as far back as I can remember. There were often times I would suddenly think of a person I hadn't heard from in a long time, and no doubt in no time at all I would get a call from that person. That was synchronicity. Think back in your own life. Did this happen to you too?

Keith passed away. You've read the story. Next, there was no funeral, but there was the drive-in burial at the cemetery. Then we moved my nephew to his new apartment. That was all done. The following day, I remained swamped because there was much to find in our papers and files. So, I spent lots of time in the office.

It was the middle of the afternoon, and I found my way down to the bedroom for something, and I stopped at the doorway. I held onto the door opening and stared at the room. Something on the end table got my full attention. I stared at the light. The lamp next to my side of the bed. The light was ON bright (there are three settings)! I stared at it, not believing it. Then, at the same time, I was thinking, "Well, let me be logical. I left the light on and can't remember it?" I have brain fog, after all. Or so I told myself. "Hmmm," I said to myself. The lights-on incidents had not happened since 2010, and it was then 2020. A whole ten years had passed. And, yes, I still had and used the same lamps.

The next day came, and it was the middle of the afternoon, and I passed by the open bedroom once again. I happened to glance inside the room. Again, I stopped in my tracks. That time my hand went to my open mouth, and I said out loud, "Oh My God. " I realized then and there that someone was contacting me. As I stood at the door, I asked out loud, "So how do I know it's Rudy or Keith?" I didn't get an answer then, but I would at another time. Surprisingly!

The lights kept turning on that particular lamp (next to my side of the bed) often for the next week or so (seemingly always in the middle of the afternoon). And then stopped. It was comforting to get the constant signs. I wondered if Rudy was letting me know Keith arrived and he was fine. Or was it Keith who had figured out the whole contact thing himself? Had he hooked up with Rudy? What were they telling each other about me? That would make for an exciting talk among two guys I had married. Would they talk about wanting to help everyone? Would they talk about the sex? I was hoping that they weren't comparing notes!

I continued my days of going through paperwork and then getting rid of more of Keith's clothes. At some time, I think I mentioned to a couple we knew that I needed to get rid of Keith's clothes. It had been a cleansing of the house that I learned about back with Rudy's death. The need to get rid of the decedent's clothes as soon as possible after death.

So, as suddenly as I thought about it again, I got a call from the couple, and they found their way to our home. Now, this is COVID-19 virus time. So, I had to be picky and careful letting anyone in the house. But I needed this masked couple's help with the clothes, so I let them in, and we were careful.

Contact...again

ON THE DAY THIS LOVELY couple came to help me with the clothes, the lady used the front restroom as they were preparing to leave. After they left, I went into the same bathroom a short time later, even though I rarely used that restroom, and found the hot water flowing. I didn't think anything of it and thought out loud, "Lady, ya left the hot water on!" After washing my hands, I said to myself, "I must make sure I turn this hot water off since I don't want to leave it on as she did."

It was many hours later, after I had used another bathroom since I used the front bathroom. So, I hadn't been in the front restroom for maybe six hours. It must have been about ten thirty p.m. when I entered the front bathroom. I came to a screeching stop as soon as I moved the door to the fully open position. I stared intently at the scene.

There before me, the hot water faucet was on full blast! I was taken aback by the view! The entirely steamed wall of mirrors meant that the hot water had been on a long time. I would have likely screamed if there had been writing on the steamed mirrors. No writing. Right then and there, I knew that Keith did this!

Later on, I would speak with the lady I'd thought left the hot water running the first time when she used the restroom, and she assured me that she never used hot water to wash her hands.

Yes, I was thoroughly convinced it was Keith that had contacted me. How did I know? Because when Keith was alive, every morning and every night while brushing his teeth in the bathroom, he would turn on the hot water full blast to keep the pipes clear and unclogged. He would do this every day for as long as I can remember, even when he was ill and could barely stand up.

Plus, remember Keith was a high-rise engineer. He was a master at electrical, air conditioning, plumbing, locksmith. You name it, and he did it with great skill and knew a thing or two.

Yes, that was Keith that had contacted me. It had been a few weeks since I got to day forty-two when I wrote that section. I hadn't witnessed the hot water on again (in the bathroom), but I did see the light on in the bedroom the week afterward. I think Keith wanted to let me know that I was heading in the right direction with all the paperwork I had to do after his death and taking care of business. I felt overwhelmed with so much to handle and I kept asking Keith for guidance in the right direction.

I had that sense. The sense that Keith was here with me, but then he wasn't. He must have been a busy angel. Because I think he had to be someone special for God in Heaven. Perhaps with all the illnesses and deaths from the COVID-19 virus, God needed more angels to help people through their grief. No doubt Keith would make an awesome angel.

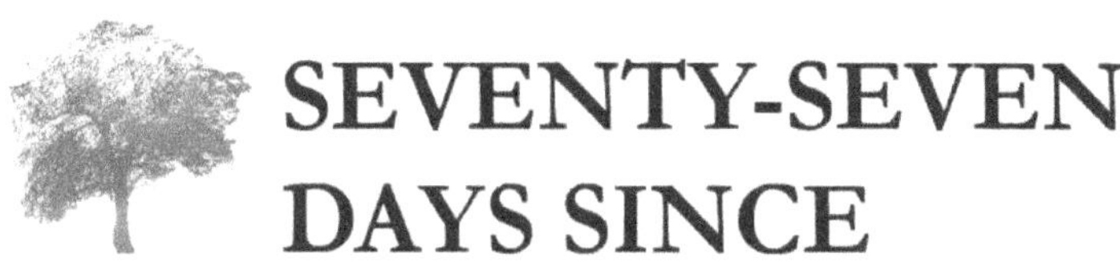# SEVENTY-SEVEN DAYS SINCE

It was Thursday, June 11, 2020. Seventy-seven days since Keith was suddenly no more. Seventy-seven days since I last kissed my husband, spoke to him, and said goodbye even though he had already left his body—seventy-seven days since I lay next to him and held his soft hand for the last time. I missed Keith so very much. Incredibly, my heart and whole person continued to ache for him.

I filled my time keeping busy, taking care of all the business needed after someone passes away. There just seemed to be an endless list to take care of, and each time I thought I'd finished or accomplished something, there would be something else needed or a new item that needed to be added to another list.

I was still in shock about Keith's demise. However, my foggy brain and numb feelings had waned a bit. Wonder remained, and even denial and disbelief that Keith had died and was gone still haunted me. How could he be gone? After all, he was supposed to live forever—he was my Superman!

The excruciating, unbearable, crushing feelings of loss had

diminished, but I still found feelings of grief returning to me, with waves of intense sorrow taking over for a few minutes here and there. Suddenly, without warning, a memory or thought would come to my mind and provoke sudden sadness, the nose tingled, tightening of the throat, stifling of the tears, crying, then bawling commenced.

It had been a while since I had reviewed the well-known "Five Stages of Grief," so I thought I would check out where I was in the grief process. I found out from past experiences that knowing, learning, and understanding the course could assist in the healing process. After studying to see where I was, I figured that I was going through them all right then. All at once!

Interestingly enough, Since Elisabeth Kübler-Ross' book *On Death and Dying* was published in 1969, which is about the Five Stages of Grief, many writers, experts in their fields, have published multiple publications expanding on the subject. These authors mentioned seven, eight, and even twelve stages of grief. The twelve stages I remembered were: shock and denial, pain and guilt, anger and bargaining, depression and reflection and loneliness, upward turn, reconstruction (working through), and finally, acceptance.

Even after a time, acceptance was not there for me. I kept catching myself saying and thinking in "WE" terms, as if Keith was still here.

Still, the shock and limbo feeling continued. Indeed, I felt I saw my husband's death coming. But did I realize it was happening? I don't know. The memory is a slow-motion collision of too many senses to give any realization about the situation. Life changes instantly, even when you think you know how it will turn out.

It was hard not to have guilt feelings all over the board. Guilt–that I did not have the hospice nurse order morphine early enough, even though Keith didn't want to go on morphine at all. He would not have been in such misery. Guilt—that I pushed Keith to keep going when he should've said enough is enough. But Keith was not a quitter, and neither was I. I still felt guilty. I'm told by friends not to feel that way but, but, but if only.

At that time, depression was just the way. But sometimes, I was neutral. Neither happy nor sad. Somewhere in between. Perhaps back in the foggy layer where my on-hold feelings existed. That was the time when I hid myself in movies or shows on TV or good ole Netflix to the rescue for binge-watching. Shows and films took me on trips with others and placed me elsewhere, sometimes far away.

I kept the little, brown, mushy, cuddlable, stuffed bear sitting next to me on our comfortable couch as I watched TV. I reached for a hug often. The bear came from the hospice company. A rosy red heart was placed strategically on its chest with Keith's name embroidered on it. Hugs with Keith Bear were the only hugs I was allowed. It was COVID-19 time, after all.

Continuing going down the list of grief stages, I liked to say that I sometimes felt like what they refer to as an "upward turn." That is, adjusting my life without Keith with a calmer time and getting more organized. That's me. I had always hated disorganization. The other day I got up earlier than usual and set about cleaning almost the entire house.

Well, one story of the home. There are two stories, and I had one to go. But that day, I was focused the whole day and was thankful with a sense of satisfaction at the end of the cleaning day that I had accomplished the task. I couldn't remember the last time I had cleaned the house. I had been putting it off with no enthusiasm.

Keith and I used to band together as our own cleaning crew. We balked when others said they had their hired cleaning crew to clean their home. We could still do it ourselves and would clean till we died. We both loved to do this together to attain the satisfaction of a clean, orderly home. Since Keith's demise, I have been the one-person cleaning crew.

Now, I found myself speaking with a friend yesterday about reinventing myself. I had mentioned reinventing myself to several friends. But I had not given it much thought, more than just saying the words. Now, as a matter of fact, I had found more than just thoughts associated with those words. Planning for the future and reconstruction is supposed to be the last step of working through Grief.

But, still, I was working through all the phases of Depression and Sorrow. Maybe not one-by-one but jumbled all together and here and there. Just like our thoughts sometimes.

I still couldn't bring myself to turn the car radio on for "our" music while driving to errands. Keith and I had our favorite music playing while in his car. Usually, the dance music of the '20s, '30s, '40s. Dance music that we both loved. But now, I rarely played any music in the car or at home. From past experience, I knew that certain music could be triggering. I turned on the small stereo in the dining room the other day while I cleaned the house. I had classical music flowing through the house the whole day, and it felt right. It didn't make me sad. I'm afraid to hear our favorite music as I know it will remind me of our dances with my beloved Keith or remind me of something else and once again make me sad. I avoided that music.

THE ONE-HUNDREDTH DAY

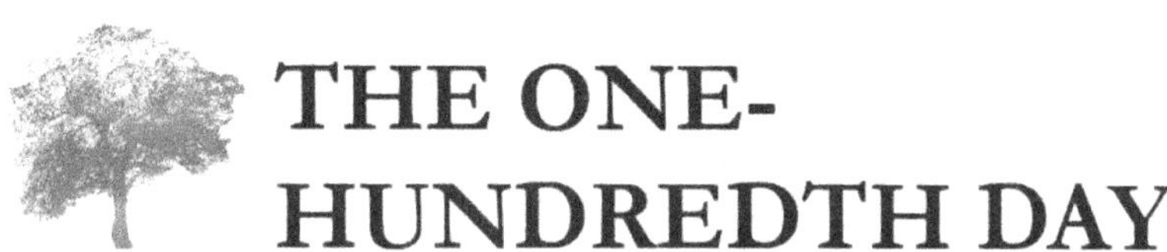

It was July 2, 2020, a Thursday. In several days it would reach the 100th—one-hundredth day since Keith's passing. Last week was pretty challenging since it marked three months, plus this past Monday marked what would have been his seventy-first birthday.

My dear Keith, how I missed you so much. My heart continued to sting from the loss of your physical being. There was never a day that went by that I didn't find instances of many wet tears seeing their way from my eyes and rolling down my cheeks. But it was my loss, not yours. Because I know you were with me when I needed you spiritually.

Some people say things like, "Well, you know Keith is always with you." I didn't feel that. Not always. I believed that in the beginning, after the spirit left the body, the spirit of Keith lingered on mainly because the spirit was trying to get bearings and figure things out. It was all new to him, the spirit world. Maybe. But after a bit of time, the spirit moved on to venture further, visit relatives, Heaven, and the universe.

Additionally, I felt that he might let me know he was around when the spirit stays around for a while. The spirit might give you signs such as sending birds to your windows, butterflies in the garden more than usual, giving off aromas such as certain colognes, cigarette or cigar smells, turning on or flickering lights, or opening water faucets. Keith had sent hummingbirds to the large kitchen window by the patio (where they rarely went), and Keith had done the last two: lights on and faucets on. He most likely learned the light trick himself. But if he didn't figure it out himself, he had help from my previous husband, Rudy.

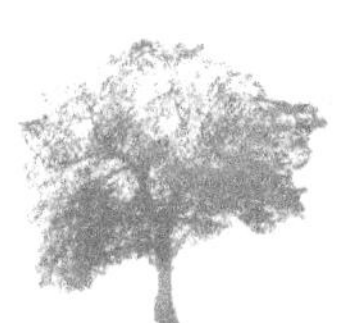

117 DAYS SINCE

This day was July 21, 2020. One hundred seventeen days since Keith died. It seemed like it just happened, and no time had elapsed.

The night before last, I had a tough time going to sleep. I was so very sleepy at the usual time. So, I closed down the TV, lights, set the alarm, and got ready for bed. Ahhh! I slipped into "our" super-soft, nice, cozy bed. Alone! Alone! ALONE!

Anger entered my once-sleepy mind, awakening it sharply. I was enraged with fury and felt sorry for myself because Keith was not there with me. Lying there flat on my back with my arms outside the covers, I pounded the bed with my clenched tight fists. Yelling at the void in the room, I kept saying, "No friggin' fair! Damn, Damn, Damn!"

Then, as usual, the yelling resolved into solitary tears. I felt so isolated, so totally alone. I couldn't see any friends and Keith was gone. The damn pandemic just kept going badly, and everyone had to stay away from everyone. It was brutal.

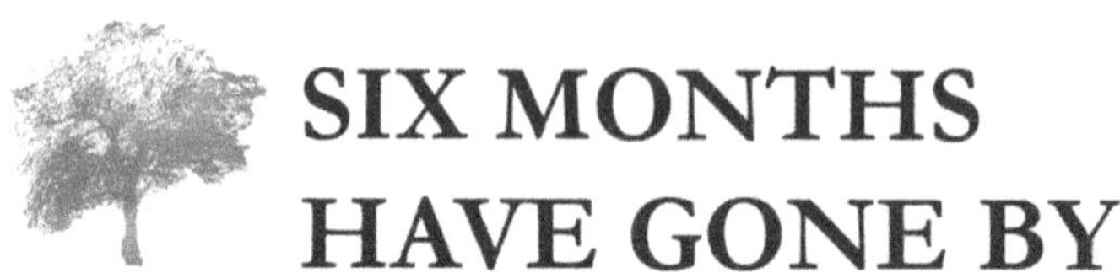# SIX MONTHS HAVE GONE BY

It was September 26, 2020, and usually, around the "twenties" days of the month, I felt that the 26th was nearing. The 26th, the day my husband died. It had then been six months. Thankfully, I believed the brain fog had released its stronghold on me, and I had more days and times of more clear and detailed thoughts again.

Although my brain fog was sometimes lifting, I still experienced the numbing effect of paralyzing spells. I grasped at the times I could think fully and clearly and tried to accomplish needed work. On top of that, I had problems seeing with one eye. Suffering from Aged Macular Degeneration had not been easy.

I needed injections once every four weeks like clockwork just to keep the degeneration at a slower pace and keep my vision. I heard some people only have to have these injections every few months or even less frequently. I long for, and I pray for this for me. The injections are not only painful in the eye, but the whole body has a physical reaction, and I am down for the count the day I have these injections. But I am grateful. I am thankful that an injection can help me continue seeing, driving, drawing, writing, and working.

Yes, I still longed for my husband. I longed to hold his hand as I fell to sleep. I caught myself still wanting to tell him something I found out but realizing he wasn't here to tell. I told him out loud anyway, thinking he might hear it in the spirit world.

As you might recall, Keith and I always had our custom to be sure we kissed and said "I Love You" to each other any time we parted or before going to sleep.

I keep a piece of Keith next to my bed. Each morning I pick it up and kiss it and talk to Keith, saying, "Good morning, I love you, Keith." I keep it in this little dark box sitting close to my eyeglass case. The golden beguiled band sits there pretty in the white cushioning inserts of the box.

Usually, I would rise from my bed each morning, and the first thing I would do was place my glasses on my face. I would then see the beautiful ring sitting pretty in the box before me. Seeing the ring always reminded me of my dear husband. I would pick up and kiss Keith's manly wedding band, and replace it back into the box. When I returned the glasses to the hard-shell protective eye glass case in the evening, I once again would lift the ring out of the box, kiss the band, and often said, "Good Night, Keith" or "I love you," place the ring back into the box, and climb into bed. That had been my homage, my ritual for my love of Keith. Forever missed.

This ritual I started just after Keith passed away. It served me well to continue the practice and continue to honor my beloved husband significantly. I know there will be a day when I decide to close up the box and put it away or do something else with the wedding band lying inside. But not in the near future.

My rituals got me through this whole mess—the mess of losing a husband. A husband I still loved immensely and grieved totally. Making matters a lot worse was the fact that the hundredth-year COVID-19 virus pandemic hit simultaneously, making everything off-limits, including cemeteries, funerals, churches, schools, malls, restaurants, beaches, gyms, movies, seeing friends, and more. Worst of all affected by the pandemic was that the much-needed hugs were banned! Handshakes gone. Masks were mandatory (as they should've been), and everyone had to take care just to go outside.

Forward I moved, as I kept telling myself each day, as they say, one day at a time, one step at a time. As I worked on this book, the story of my Superman husband, Keith, I knew I had a life ahead that would be very different from my life with Keith. I'm writing my own new life story since I must reinvent myself. Will I dance again? I pondered this, especially in the throes of the COVID-19 pandemic restricting gathering and, yes, prohibiting dancing. I realized my friends were all dance friends since we spent so much time dancing. Finding real friends then was both critical and extremely hard to accomplish. Finding new friends was impossible. It was a tough time all around.

Back before Christmas of 2020, I placed Keith's ring back into its box and hid it away for protection. I know the vows say, "until death do us part." But I was not ready to end my connection to my dear husband. I continued to wear my wedding rings on my wedding finger. I had never removed the rings since we married in 2003 except for cleaning. They still sparkled and were a constant reminder of our deep love together. Now and forever.

Almost a year later, on March 27, 2021, we were finally able to hold a proper funeral church service for Keith! One year and one day after Keith passed away, I pressed our local church and its priest along with another of Keith's favorite priests (the one who presided over his tiny burial) to preside at Keith's memorial mass. Since COVID restraints still bound us, I could only have seventy-five people attend the outdoor mass (COVID-19 protocol only allowing outdoor services). Those of importance to Keith attended. A few even traveled from far away to be there for the service. I was very thankful everyone was well enough to attend.

We were all masked and staying the distance, and alas, still no hugs were allowed (but very much on my mind as my body ached for hugs). Thankfully, the service was outside under a large wooden pavilion at the local church. It was a beautiful and meaningful service with both priests speaking kindly about Keith plus thankfully great music.

For the past year, I had felt as though I was waiting to exhale and take that next step but could not because the service for Keith had not happened. For me, it was a great release and send-off for my loving Keith. Now I could rest, and I felt Keith then able to go on with his new spirit adventures.

"Goodbye, my shining bright prince. Goodbye, my Superman. I kiss your perfectly smooth gold wedding ring and turn off the lamp. Good night, my dearest and magnificent husband. Au Revoir. Adieu!"

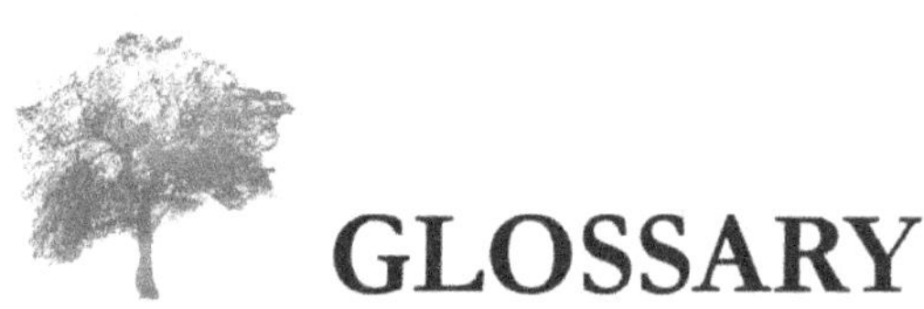

GLOSSARY

5FU: Fluorouracil

5FU is a chemotherapy drug that slows the growth of cancer cells. 5FU, as it is often called, is used in conjunction with other targeting chemotherapies or antibodies or sometimes alone.

Advocacy

"Patient advocacy is an area of specialization in health care concerned with advocacy for patients, survivors, and caregivers. The patient advocate may be an individual or an organization, often, though not always, concerned with one specific group of disorders." Per Wikipedia. (Read the Advocacy section for more information)

Aortic valve replacement

"When the aortic valve isn't working properly, it can interfere with blood flow and force the heart to work harder to send blood to the rest of your body. Aortic valve repair or aortic valve replacement can treat aortic valve disease and help restore normal blood flow, reduce symptoms, prolong life, and help preserve the function of your heart muscle." Per Mayoclinic.org. Check this link for more information–

https://www.mayoclinic.org/tests-procedures/aortic-valve-repair-aortic-valve-replacement/about/pac-20385093

Avastin

Avastin is a tumor-starving (anti-angiogenic) therapy. Avastin is used to block the protein, VEGF– Vascular endothelial growth factor. Designed to work with chemotherapy to prevent tumor growth. Read more

https://www.avastin.com/patient/mcrc/about/how-avastin-works.html

BRCA2

BRCA2 is the cancer-fighting gene that works to keep cancer away. "Tumor suppressor proteins help prevent cells from growing and dividing too rapidly or in an uncontrolled way." See more at this link–

https://medlineplus.gov/genetics/gene/brca2/

(Read more in the section HER2 and BRCA2 in this book)

Cancer History

https://www.cancer.org/treatment/understanding-your-diagnosis/history-of-cancer/what-is-cancer.html

CDC

https://www.cdc.gov/cancer/breast/young_women/bringyourbrave/hereditary_breast_cancer/index.htm

CEA

Carcinoembryonic antigen. Better known as a tumor marker acronym. High numbers may indicate certain cancers such as colon, rectum, prostate, ovary, lung, thyroid, or liver.

CPR

Cardiopulmonary Resuscitation. Emergency lifesaving treatment used when heart stops beating. Fast help with CPR can save a person's life. Learn more at this link

https://cpr.heart.org/en/resources/what-is-cpr

Chemotherapy infusions

Chemotherapy drugs pushed thru a catheter that is inserted in a vein or artery. Chemotherapy is often infused via PICC-lines or port-a-cath devices.

C-line

C-line or central line is a venous line placed into the large vein. (Read more about the C-line in the Liver Lobectomy section)

Colostomy

A surgical operation in which a part of the colon is diverted to an opening through the body to the outside (making an ostomy) to bypass a bad or damaged part of the colon. The damaged colon area is either repaired to removed. Often the colon is surgically placed together in a later surgery (usually months later to allow internal healing of damaged areas). A Colostomy bag is attached to the outside of the body to catch the bodily defecations.

Comptosar

Irinotecan. "Considered an anti-cancer chemotherapy drug. Classified as a "plant alkaloid" and "topoisomerase I inhibitor." Read more at this link–

https://chemocare.com/chemotherapy/drug-info/camptosar.aspx

Cryoablation

A needle is inserted thru the skin into the tumor area and the tumor is treated with extreme cold to freeze the tumor. (Read more in the Cryoablation section). Check out the link below–

https://www.mayoclinic.org/tests-procedures/cryoablation-for-cancer/about/pac-20385216#:~:text=Cryoablation%20for%20cancer%20is%20a,tissue%20is%20allowed%20to%20thaw

CT scan

"Ct is a diagnostic imaging procedure that uses a combination of x-rays and computer technology to produce images of the inside of the body." Read more at this link–

https://www.hopkinsmedicine.org/health/treatment-tests-and-therapies/computed-tomography-ct-scan#:~:text=A%20CT%20scan%20is%20a%20diagnostic%20imaging%20procedure%20that%20uses,detailed%20than%20standard%20X%2Drays.

CVA

Cerebrovascular accident. "A loss of blood flow to part of the brain, which damages brain tissue. CVA's are caused by blood clots and broken vessels in the brain." Read more at this link

https://www.cancer.gov/publications/dictionaries/cancer-terms/def/cva

ERCP

Endoscopic retrograde cholangiopancreatography. A procedure

to diagnose and treat problems in the liver, gallbladder, bile ducts, and pancreas. (Read more in the ERCP section)

www.hopkinsmedicine.org:

https://www.hopkinsmedicine.org/health/treatment-tests-and-therapies/endoscopic-retrograde-cholangiopancreatography-ercp

Fentanyl

A narcotic/synthetic opioid. 80-100 times stronger than morphine. Developed for treatment for pain management for cancer patients in patch form.

Genentech

Major pharmaceutical company that produced the DNA HER2 testing and producing the subsequent monoclonal antibody drugs, Herceptin and Perjeta.

Genomic DNA Testing

"Genomic testing is often confused with genetic testing. The main difference is that genetic tests are designed to detect a single gene mutation (such as the BRCA1 and BRCA2 mutations associated with breast and ovarian cancer), while genomic tests look at all of your genes." Read more at this link

https://www.gene.com/stories/getting-personal-with-genomics

Heart Math

https://www.heartmath.org/

HER2

Usually seen in connection with breast cancer or gastric and gastroesophageal cancer. Human epidermal growth factor receptor 2. Cancer fighting gene that works to keep cancer away. When HER2 goes into hyperactivity metabolically, they become cancer-producing genes instead. (Read more about HER2 in the section HER2 and BRCA2)

Hemorrhagic Stroke

"A hemorrhagic stroke occurs when blood from an artery suddenly begins bleeding into the brain. As a result, the part of the body controlled by the damaged area of the brain cannot work properly." Read more at this link–

https://www.cedars-sinai.org/health-library/diseases-and-conditions/h/hemorrhagic-stroke.html#:~:text=A%20hemorrhagic%20stroke%20occurs%20when,bleeding%20occurs%20inside%20the%20brain

Hemothorax

An accumulation of blood and fluid in pleural cavity commonly caused by chest trauma. But percutaneous insertion thru the skin and thru the chest wall for RFA (radio frequency ablation) can also be a causal factor. Read more at this link–

https://www.ncbi.nlm.nih.gov/books/NBK538219/

Herceptin

Trastuzumab. Monoclonal antibody treatment used in combination with Perjeta for breast cancer HER2 and BRCA2. (Read more in the Perjeta and Herceptin section)

Hospice

Care for a person nearing the end of life that includes good quality of life as possible with as much comfort as possible. Usually for those whose disease cannot be controlled and soon will end the person's life. All curing attempts have stopped due to failures. Read more about hospice at the National Institute of Aging website below:

Hypermetabolic activity

Excessive surge in metabolic rate. Cancer falls into the category hypermetabolic. However, inflammation and infection can also be in the hypermetabolic state. So, it is important to get a doctor to figure which is which.

https://connect.mayoclinic.org/discussion/oakhillbull/

KRAS

KRAS is a gene known as oncogenes. If mutated, KRAS have potential of causing regular cells to turn cancerous. There is much more information in the link below.

https://medlineplus.gov/genetics/gene/kras/

https://www.cancer.gov/publications/dictionaries/cancer-terms/def/wild-type-kras-gene

Leucovorin

An antidote to bad effects of cancer medicines given in high doses. Given to prevent anemia. Works like folic acid which also may be low in patients undergoing heavy duty cancer treatment.

https://www.mayoclinic.org/drugs-supplements/leucovorin-oral-route-intravenous-route-injection-route/description/drg-20064503#:~:text=Leucovorin%20is%20used%20as%20an,be%20low%20in%20these%20patients.

Liver ablation

Most ablations can be done by inserting a needle into the skin and then into the targeted tumor. Types of ablations are RFA (radiofrequency ablation), MWA (microwave ablation), and Cryoablation (freezing the tumor).

https://www.cancer.org/cancer/liver-cancer/treating/tumor-ablation.html#:~:text=Ablation%20is%20treatment%20that%20destroys,health%20or%20reduced%20liver%20function).

Liver Lobectomy

Removal of one lobe of the liver leaving the remainder of the liver to take over all operations of the liver. (Read more in the Liver Lobectomy section)

MDAnderson

https://www.mdanderson.org/cancerwise/tai-chi-healing-from-the-inside-out.h00-158598468.html

MRI

Magnetic resonance imaging. Detailed images of the anatomy (organs and tissues) generated by computer-generated radio waves. Read more about MRI at this link:

https://www.mayoclinic.org/tests-procedures/mri/about/pac-20384768#:~:text=Magnetic%20resonance%20imaging%20(MRI)%20is,large%2C%20tube%2Dshaped%20magnets.

MRI Stroke Staging

https://radiopaedia.org/articles/haemorrhage-on-mri?lang=us

New Thought Movement

https://www.newthoughtwisdom.com/about-new-thought.html

Oncologist

Doctor specializing in the diagnosing and treating of cancer. Read in-depth info at this link:

https://www.webmd.com/a-to-z-guides/what-is-an-oncologist

Ostomy

Surgery to make a new opening for wastes to leave the body when the colon, intestine, rectum, or bladder fail. Stoma is the name of the opening. Sometimes it is permanent and sometimes the operation is reversed after the area that was operated on is healed. Look at this link for more info:

https://medlineplus.gov/ostomy.html

Oxaliplatin

Type of chemotherapy for bowel and other cancers. This chemotherapy drug stops the development of the DNA and eradicates the cancer cell. Check this link for more info

https://www.cancerresearchuk.org/about-cancer/cancer-in-general/treatment/cancer-drugs/drugs/oxaliplatin-eloxatin#:~:text=Oxaliplatin%20is%20a%20type%20of,drugs%20you%20have%20it%20with.

PBD/IR

Cholangiogram transhepatic. Percutaneous biliary drainage (PBD) Interventional radiology. (Read more in the PBD/IR section)

https://www.hopkinsmedicine.org/interventional-radiology/procedures/pctpbd/

Perjeta

Pertuzumab. Monoclonal antibody treatment used in combination with Perjeta for breast cancer HER2 and BRCA2. (Read more in the Perjeta and Herceptin section)

PET scan

Positron emission tomography. Uses radioactive radiotracers to measure metabolic or biochemical activity of tissues and organs. Cancer is often detected on this test before others such as CAT/CT/MRI. Read more at this link:

https://www.mayoclinic.org/tests-procedures/pet-scan/about/pac-20385078

PICC line

A PICC line is a small tube that they put inside a large vein in your arm, and it goes all the way to your heart, where the liquid is pumped throughout your body without destroying your veins.

Pneumothorax

"A pneumothorax occurs when air leaks into the space between your lung and chest wall. This air pushes on the outside of your lung and makes it collapse." Per Mayoclinic.org.

https://www.mayoclinic.org/diseases-conditions/pneumothorax/symptoms-causes/syc-20350367

Port-a-cath

A piece of equipment that is inserted under the skin and guided into a large vein above the right side of the heart (superior vena cava). Port-o-cath's are using for intravenous transfusions, antibiotics, drawing blood, and chemotherapy infusions. Read more at this link

https://www.cancer.gov/publications/dictionaries/cancer-terms/def/port-a-cath

Qigong

"Qigong is a centuries-old system of coordinated body posture and movement, breathing, and meditation used for the purposes of health, spirituality, and martial arts training." Per Wikipedia. (Read more in Qigong section)

Quadruple bypass surgery

Redirects blood around blocked artery section in the heart. Healthy blood vessels are removed from other parts of the body and connected making new improved flow to the heart muscle. Read more at this link:

https://www.mayoclinic.org/tests-procedures/coronary-bypass-surgery/about/pac-20384589

Resect colon/Colectomy

Bowel resection surgery. A piece of the affected colon is removed in surgery. Read more at this link:

https://my.clevelandclinic.org/health/treatments/4671-colectomy-bowel-resection-surgery

Percutaneous

Thru the skin. Via needle puncture.

Perjeta

https://www.perjeta.com/patient/how-perjeta-works.html?c=per-16e8fec5ef8&gclid=CjwKCAiAtouOBhA6EiwA2nLKH4X5je8F08RugGSUSUwTlucF0Zah6UFKQhP2B8ymtDM_flbcQ_2RDhoCnLgQAvD_BwE&gclsrc=aw.ds

RFA

Radiofrequency ablation. Read more about RFA in the RFA Ablation section.

https://www.radiologyinfo.org/en/info/rfaliver

Sloan-Kettering Cancer Center: Nausea

https://www.mskcc.org/cancer-care/patient-education/acupressure-nausea-and-vomiting

Stroke

https://www.ahajournals.org/doi/10.1161/STROKEAHA.119.027198

Tama-do

Sound and color healing. (Read more in the Tama-do section)

Tai-chi

"Tai chi, short for T'ai chi ch'üan or Tàijíquán, is an internal Chinese martial art practiced for defense training, health benefits, and meditation. Tai chi has practitioners worldwide." Per Wikipedia. (Read more in our Tai-Chi section)

Tai-chi Vs Structured Exercise

https://www.clinicaltrials.gov/ct2/show/NCT00246818

Thoracentesis

Process to remove excess fluid in the space between the lungs and chest wall (pleural effusions).

Tao-te-Ching

https://www.britannica.com/topic/Tao-te-Ching

Tumor marker

Doctors use tumor marker tests to learn if someone has cancer. There are different tumor marker tests for many types of cancers. Read more at this link:

https://www.cancer.net/navigating-cancer-care/diagnosing-cancer/tests-and-procedures/tumor-marker-tests

UCLA-Power of Positivity Study

https://exploreim.ucla.edu/mind-body/power-of-positivity/

Vectibix

Panitumumab. Used along with other chemotherapy treatments for wild-type KRAS metastatic cancer. Read more at this link:

https://www.vectibix.com/?isipaid=true&gclid=CjwKCAjws8y UBhA1EiwAi_tpEc2LCRIiNA8omeG0UEIUGSAJJ9VIINX6TbnE HIPymmtHj8xSuho4NxoCM-IQAvD_BwE&gclsrc=aw.ds

Y90 Yttrium radioactive beads

Tiny radioactive beads injected directly to the blood supply to the tumor and sometimes directly into the tumor itself. Other vessels have temporary blocks placed so that the beads do not stray into other areas that can be greatly affected. Read more at this link:

https://www.columbiaradiology.org/patients/services/interventio nal-radiology/y90-treatment-radioembolization

Xeloda

Capecitabine. Given in pill form Pills taken 3 in the morning and 3 in the evening. Treatment for colon, rectum, and breast cancer. Read more at this link:

https://www.gene.com/patients/medicines/xeloda

Zaltrap

Zaltrap is an antineoplastic and VEGF (vascular endothelial growth factor). Used in connection with other chemotherapy for the treatment of metastatic colorectal cancer. Read more at this link:

https://chemocare.com/chemotherapy/drug-info/zaltrap.aspx

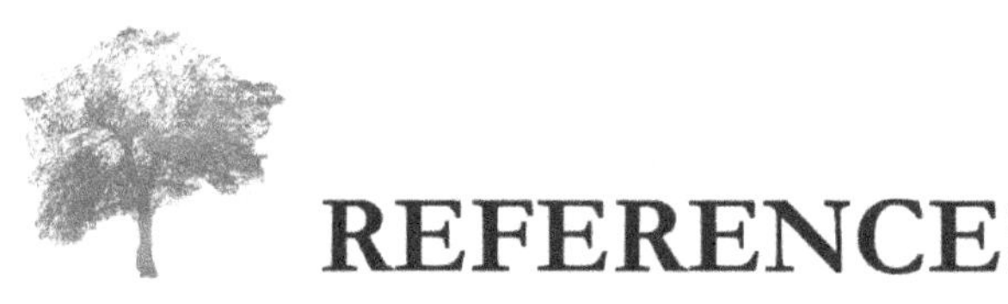

REFERENCES

A Spiritual Path for Spiritual Living. https://www.unityofcitrus.org/qigong

Bhajan, Yogi. https://www.goodreads.com/quotes/95446-an-attitude-of-gratitude-brings-great-things

Buddha. https://sourcesofinsight.com/buddha-quotes/

Byrne, Rhonda. *The Secret.* New York, London, Toronto, Sydney, New Delhi. Atria Books. Hillsboro, Oregon. Beyond Words Publishing. 2005.

Byrne, Rhonda. *The Greatest Secret.* New York, NY: HarperOne, an imprint of HarperCollins Publishers. 2020.

Byrne, Rhonda. *The Secret to Health Masterclass.* New York, NY: Simon and Schuster Audio. 2020.

Braden, Gregg. https://www.heartmath.org/

Chopra, Deepak. *Ageless Body, Timeless Mind: The Quantum Alternative to Growing Old.* New York: Harmony Books. 1993.

Dyer, Dr. Wayne. *The Power of Intention.* Hay House. 2010.

Dyer, Dr. Wayne, *You Are What You Think*. Facebook Calendar Faith Affirming. www.waynedyer.com

Gawande, Atul. *Being Mortal: Medicine and What Matters in the End.* Picador. 175 Fifth Avenue. New York, NY 10010. 2014.

Golter, Samuel. https://www.cityofhope.org/about-city-of-hope/who-we-are

Guex,Patrice, translated by Heather Goodare. *An Introduction to Psycho-oncology*. Routledge. London and New York. 1994.

Guthrie, Nancy. *The One Year Book of Hope.* Tyndale Momentum. Tyndale House Publishers Inc. Carol Stream, Illinois. 2005.

Hay, Louise L. https://www.louisehay.com/forgiveness/

Hay, L.L. *You Can Heal Your Life*. Santa Monica, CA. Hay House. 1987.

Hill, Napoleon. *Think and Grow Rich*. Original 1937. Shippensburg, PA: Sound Wisdom Publishing.2016

Holy Bible/King James Version. 1 Corinthians 13:1-8,13/ Philippians 4:13/Matthew 26:38

Jefferson, Thomas. Quote: "Important truths; that knowledge is power, knowledge is safety and knowledge is happiness." 1817 Letter.

Marley, Bob. https://www.goodreads.com/quotes/884474-you-never-know-how-strong-you-are-until-being-strong

https://en.wikipedia.org/wiki/New_Thought

https://en.wikipedia.org/wiki/Positive_Thinking

Mayo Clinic. https://www.mayoclinic.org/healthy-lifestyle/stress-management/in-depth/positive-thinking/art-20043950

MD Anderson Cancer Center. https://www.mdanderson.org/cancerwise/tai-chi-healing-from-the-inside-out.h00-158598468.html

Mukherjee, M.D., Siddhartha. *The Emperor of All Maladies. A*

Biography of Cancer. Scribner, A Division of Simon & Schuster, Inc. 1230 Avenue of the Americas. New York, NY 10020. 2010.

NCBI (National Center for Biotechnology Information). https://www.ncbi.nlm.nih.gov/pmc/articles/PMC5597070/

Nietzsche, Friedrich. https://news.northwestern.edu/stories/2019/10/science-proves-that-what-doesnt-kill-you-makes-you-stronger/

Peale, Dr. Norman Vincent. *The Power of Positive Thinking*. London. England: Cedar Books. 1990.

Robbins, Tony. https://www.tonyrobbins.com/positive-thinking/

Schuller, Robert H. *Tough Times Never Last, But Tough People Do*! Nashville. T. Nelson Publishers. 1983.

Tama-do. https://tama-do.com

UCLA. https://exploreim.ucla.edu/mind-body/power-of-positivity/

U. S. National Library of Medicine. *Effect of Tai Chi vs. structured exercise on physical fitness and stress in cancer survivors.* https://www.clinicaltrials.gov/ct2/show/NCT00246818

www.CaringBridge.com

Wark, Chris. 2020. *Beat Cancer Daily*. Hay House, Inc. www.hayhouse.com. Carlsbad, California. New York City. London. Sydney. New Delhi.